NEVER ENOUGH

HOW A DIET QUEEN LEARNED TO LOVE HERSELF
& EAT LIKE A NORMAL PERSON

KELLY FISHER

Published by KELLY FISHER / THE PRIMAL BEING
ISBN 978-0-244-43004-7

Contents

A MASSIVE, HEARTFELT, THANKS

TO MY DEAREST MUM AND DAD

I seriously could not have asked for
better parents.
Cliché as it sounds, you have given me
the best parts of yourselves.
This has made me the person I am.
The person I am proud of.

The love, attention, kindness, and caring
I received growing up, is what has made
me a <u>fighter</u>.
Even in my times of despair, I have known
there is better out there.
Better for me.
I would never have known this if you had
not loved me so fiercely.
By giving me love so abundantly, you
taught me to believe I deserved it. You
have made me 'love entitled'.

TO MY TREASURE, MY HUSBAND

Growing up, I knew I would always find
someone who was my equal, my best friend.
Someone passionate about me and me in
return.
Nothing prepared me for this.
John, you are everything I ever dreamed
of and so much more. You are the best man
I have ever met.
An amazing father, even when the tide is
against you.
A loving husband, even when your wife is
a little cray cray.

I have never once doubted your love for
me.
Even now years later you make me feel
like I am the only person in the room.
Even now when you don't understand some
of my hobbies, passions, and dreams, you
are my cheer squad.
Thank you for supporting me through my
journey of healing.
Something Australian Olympian Kurt
Fearnely said that stuck with me was
this: support of good people around you
is the main thing a person needs to
succeed.

I have hit the jackpot with you.

LASTLY, A WARM THANK YOU TO EVERYONE ELSE WHO HAS SUPPORTED ME

Particularly through my healing.

All it takes is a small interaction to affect a person's life.
There have been so many people who have shaped my journey, which led me to the desire to get off the diet roller coaster and start living my life.

A massive immeasurable thanks.

Chapter 1 – My Story

WHO AM I?

I am a 40-year-old woman, Step-Mummy of two great young adults and loving wife to one amazing man.
I live in Brisbane, Australia where the sun shines for 283 days of the year.
So already, this makes me *lucky*.

I have had a pretty *regular* life.
And by regular, I mean I have had good times, painful times, ups and downs.
I have been hurt, I have been loved.
I have felt on top of the world *and* like I was buried at the bottom of the sea with *what felt like* no way to gasp for air.

I am *lucky*.
Did you know here in Australia, when compared to the population of the world, we are richer than approx. 99% of the world's population?
Care International provides a calculator on their website which shows what percentage you fall in based on the income of all other people in the world. And even when I punched in the lowest average income for an Australian, we are still in the top 1%.
Yes, 99% of people in the world are poorer than us, living in conditions way worse than us.
People face crime like abduction, rape, and murder daily. Theft, little food and lack of health care is the norm in many places.

The reason I am telling you this is I don't think *my* problems are anywhere near as horrific.
BUT, we are human, and our problems, when they are

ours, are the worst thing we know.

They are the worst thing we are experiencing.

So, at that moment, when we are not looking at the big picture, our problems, are the <u>only</u> problems.

Food, which is a necessity to all human beings, food which so many people do not have access to, has been *my* worst enemy.

I am not stupid, but I sure have felt that way when I could not unravel the mystery of why it had taken over my life so deeply.

I have not understood food, I have hated it, I have loved it.

It had been drawn into a part of my life that had nothing to do with sustenance.

It had been a puzzle I was so desperate to solve and this book is a journey of what I have learned trying to figure it out.

Food had literally become my *poison*.

A PERSONAL JOURNEY

This is a story of my lifelong battle with diet obsession, eating disorders and let's face it, hating my body.

I will share everything with you, the good, bad, ugly and the most wonderful discovery that helped me with my healing once and for all. This is my fairy-tale story.

But in this story, I was my very own Prince Charming. This is a story of my roller-coaster love affair with dieting and hating myself so deeply, and finally finding my happily ever after.

I will be 100% transparent, hoping to inspire others to not make the same mistakes.

I will give you the details of everything I did and the feelings I felt along the way.

However, I guess I must warn you that what you are about to read may feel a little heavy at times. But hey, with all that extra weight on me, that is how I felt. Heavy.

Not only in my body, but in my mind.

I have lived a life consumed by trying to be better and trying to be something other than me.

I have decided to share because I am hoping to 'catch' women before they get to 40. I am hoping a 25-year-old reads this, and they are so inspired that they get off the diet roller-coaster for good and claim their life back even sooner than I did.

Hell, even if you are 70! Who wants to have a thing like dieting ruling their life forever?

I know there are many women out there who have experienced disordered eating over the years and speaking from experience, it feels oh, so shameful. The fact that I am writing this today feels like a miracle. Why a miracle? I didn't want a soul to know. I wanted to look like I had it together. I wanted to be the perfect *everything*. I didn't want to tell people I didn't know how to eat. Isn't that the first thing you learn to do? Shouldn't that just be a natural instinct?

It's shameful 'times' a million!

The reason I am sharing my story is that I hope to inspire and encourage women like me to take hold of their life and learn to love the number one person in it. Themselves.

I am horrified that we have a health system which doesn't take these issues seriously, we have body image issues causing so many people daily pain.

And for what?

WHAT MAKES ME QUALIFIED?

Ladies and Gents, this is a personal journey, I am not qualified to give you any advice.
I am not a psychologist, dietitian or doctor.

This book is not about some new 'fan-dangled' quick fix. Quite the opposite.
It has been the most wonderful self-discovery and love affair of my life.

I am a gal, just like you, who has been on the craziest of rides with health, diet, and self-esteem; this is a personal story of how I got off this merry-go-round.

I won't be telling you to follow my way or the highway. Quite the opposite.
What my journey to recovery has taught me is there are 1000's of ways to heal.
My way 'ain't' going to be your way.
What I hope to provide you is the <u>inspiration</u> and the tools that lead me to recovery.

WHAT WAS MY ISSUE?

I know I'm not super special. My issue's are no different to that of thousands of other women. There are plenty of people who look in the mirror and hate what they see and do anything they can to fix it.
But what was my *specific* 'poison'?
A combination of eating issues, disorders, possible addiction, not understanding how to deal with stress, lack of self-love and lack of self-esteem.

I mean, it makes sense when you read the stats. I was going to provide you some of those stats here, but they change so frequently, and so many sites have differing numbers so I left them out.
Suffice to say, what I saw indicated I am not alone.

So really, I'm not that special, am I?
But I wanted to be. I didn't want to be one of the statistics anymore.
To live a life hating my reflection.
I wanted to take my life back.
I wanted to be that woman so busy living life that she was not dieting at 50!

But could I do it?
And more to the point, could I give up dicting and still be healthy?

Chapter 2 – The Beginning

I guess from the minute I decided to never diet again, this became my life's work.

When I first quit diets, I didn't have a plan but out of the rubble, a plan emerged.
When I say *rubble*, I am referring to the fact that when I quit diets, I just did.
I knew morally I wanted this, so I did it. And with lack of forethought or planning of any description, I initially, made a *meal* of it. (So punny, aren't I?)

I hadn't made a plan to deal with all the other *stuff* that was going on around food and self-love (that dieting was masking all those years).

I am going to:
Take you back to where it all started
Tell you about all the things I did wrong
Share all the things I did right
Inspire and encourage you to embark on your very own journey

CHILDHOOD

I had a wonderful childhood. I look back on it and remember so many great times.
I do also remember some not so great times.
I was a *little* chubby.
I know this, not just because I have pictures to look back on, but because there were <u>many</u> people in my life who made it really clear.

My grandparents would point it out when they were

comparing my two beloved female cousins to me.
"You look pretty, but Karen is skinner than you" was a
frequent one I heard.
"You need to lose some weight," my grandmother
would say.
My aunties and uncles would also get in on the action in
more subtle ways.
Even male cousins would tease me, calling me a
tomato(because I was round. HAHA).

I remember these moments vividly because they were
painful and confusing.

I am sure nobody meant harm, *especially* the younger
cousins.
I am sure the 'oldies' were all trying to inspire me.
Perhaps they were trying to make me want to starve
myself so I could get skinny?
I am <u>sure</u> they were not trying to diminish my self-
esteem or encourage me to hide a chocolate behind the
couch so I could eat it later (which is what I would do).

THE BEGINNING OF THE END (I am such a drama
queen, right??!)

When I was about 7, I had *special* external visitors come
to my primary school.
I don't remember their qualifications, but I will guess
they were nurses or doctors.
They came into my class to perform assessments. Each
student had a turn at having their height and weight
measured to see if they were healthy.
I don't really remember the details of <u>that day</u>, but I do

remember going to the doctor with my parents a few days after, as per the school's recommendation.

My parents, being the loving people they were, jumped right onto this recommendation as they felt it was the right thing to do.
(My mum has recently told me she felt it was against what she really wanted to do, but she felt torn as she just wanted the best for me. Love you, Mum, I totally get it.)

The doctor told me I was a fatty boomba.
OK, I am exaggerating *slightly* here. I don't think that was the exact, technical term he used,
I don't remember the exact words he used, but he said I needed to lose weight.
He made me leave the room so he could talk to my parents. I don't remember what went on exactly, but I just remember from then on, being on a diet.
Looking back, I don't remember NOT being on one.

I have no huge bank of memories from back then (soooo long ago), but a couple spring to mind.
This one time at the local pool, my mum sent me to get some lunch and a drink from the canteen.
I was on a diet at the time.
I had a list of naughty foods I could not eat.
Kit-Kat *must* have been on that list because when I got back to my mum, I laid down and pulled the towel over my head… so nobody would notice I was eating said Kit-Kat.
I probably wouldn't have remembered this story had I not been sprung.
I actually don't remember buying the chocolate.
I only remember the shame of being caught red-handed.

My mum, to this day, says she felt so horrible that she listened to the doctor which had me sneaking around eating things I was not allowed to. She thought she was helping me. She says she wishes she had done things differently.
I get it. I totally get it.

When I look back, I guess I didn't understand. If I can try and recall my state, the only thing I can muster up is feelings of embarrassment, shame, guilt and not feeling good enough. I was *bad* because I was chubby.
I didn't understand why I was bad, *why* the thing I was doing wrong or *why* it was important to NOT be chubby.
I just knew I was naughty.
And being a tomato was bad.

MIXED MESSAGES

When I was 9, my parents decided to get a divorce. It was the nicest divorce in history, I am sure (no sarcasm here, I promise it was nice).

I just don't remember it being bad in the slightest.
My parents didn't love each other enough to stay married, but they loved me enough to ensure I did not feel the brunt of the divorce.
They cared more about my happiness and sustained relationship with both parents than their egos.
It wasn't until I was about 30 I discovered it was my mum's decision to get a divorce.
Until then I just thought 'Mummy and Daddy didn't love each other anymore'.
I had no blame in my mind causing me to have a lesser relationship with either parent.

When I discovered my mum instigated the divorce, I was mature enough to understand relationships and not care or judge her.

Speaking from experience with my own stepchildren, it doesn't matter how mature you think your kids are, they are still children until they have experience in adult relationships.
Watching my step kids not have what I was so lucky to have has hurt them.
This makes me understand just how blessed I was.
Not that I want anyone to get a divorce, but if you do, you need to speak to my mum & dad on how to do it best with kids.
They nailed it.

Of course, I didn't know that at the time. But looking back, and looking at the people around me now, I really couldn't have wished for a better divorce experience (if that is something you can wish for).

They sat me down to break the news about the pending divorce. They were united in their love for me, and in assuring me that life would still be great. They told me I would still get to see both my mum and dad whenever I wanted, and our houses would be close.
They both loved me very much.
I was 9, and apparently, a little shallow, because the additional announcement of having double the presents at Christmas and Birthdays sealed the deal.

I feel like what I am about to share may be construed as negative or biased towards one parent or another, but it is not intended that way. They were both 100% amazing

and anything that has happened in my life is 100% my responsibility and 100% perfect.
I see both my pain and my joy equally as important in making me the person I am.

No matter how great a divorce is, when there are two people raising a child, there are two messages. Nobody is at fault for this. It's just how it is.
When you have one household raising a child, the message is *normally* a little more consistent and there is *generally* more stability.

As I was clearly born to live the journey I have travelled, the two households were a perfect breeding ground to fertilize my eating disorder and confused relationship with food.
To many others, it may not have had an impact, but for me, it was just the fuel I needed to ignite what was already burning within me.

My Mumma Bear was uber healthy.
She was a fitness instructor by this stage and would frequent the gym daily. In fact, often, twice daily.
I recall dinners to be big salads with fish or some other protein and lots of good 'vegiful' food. <u>Lots</u>.
We had no 'junk' in the house.

My Pappa Bear was a typical Greek man. Not massive into the cooking, that's what wives are for. ;)
Going to Dad's was soooo fun. Pizza pockets, coco pops, ice cream, chips, chocolate.
A 9-year-old's heaven.
Don't get me wrong, he would make a concerted effort to give me veggies with a good dinner, but there was no

shortage of junk food in the cupboard for late night snacks and sitting and watching telly.
He made sure his place was a happy place for a 9-year-old.
He loved me (still does).

At Mum's place, we would go for walks, go to the gym, eat salad and have a treat once a fortnight.
My mum also loved me with food. I am sure she would pile on enough to feed a bodybuilder. And I ate it.
She would tell me to eat a banana because it had potassium which I needed. Or an orange because it had vitamin C. Everything was spoken about in vitamins. It wasn't food. It was nourishment.
She loved me with food too.
That's the Greek thing to do after all!

My parents are great parents.
They never ever in a million years would have known that their gift to me, generous Greek style food love, would haunt me all my life.
They were keeping their daughter fed.
Parenting basic instinct 101, right?
They did nothing wrong.
I clearly had stuff going on *upstairs,* like messages from society telling me I was not good enough. Food was merely the vehicle.

Fast forward to adulthood. The mixture of inconsistent eating, eating disorders, diets and low self-esteem that comes from being overweight had affected me.

Once you get on the diet train, it's hard to get off.
It was easy to become addicted to the buzz of momentarily looking great.

I had no intention for it to be momentary by the way.
I believed that once I lost the weight, and got out of the
mess I was in, I would be normal, <u>and</u> my stomach
would shrink <u>and</u> in turn, I would be able to eat like a
normal person.

I feel I have lived with this disease, this unhealthy
relationship with food, all my life.
Every diet I have ever gone on was stepped into with the
intention I would lose the weight and then after *the 12
weeks were over* I would be sitting pretty.

I guess that's the diet industry.
It's designed to fix you temporarily, in a time frame, to
make you lose weight and say 'Yes! It worked'.
It's my belief that diets are not designed to help you
long term with everything else that is going on with <u>you;</u>
that needs to be sorted first.
How was I supposed to know this when I was a
teenager?
When I was so desperate to look pretty for <insert
various *ever desperately important occasion* here>.

SCHOOL, LIFE AND GROWING UP

School brought another level of joy when we had sport.
I hated it!
I hated it because it meant having to get changed with all
the *skinny* girls and I was petrified they would see my
body and tease me like they teased other overweight
kids.
I was clever though, I found a great solution!
I would pretend to be sick on sport days. Smart huh?

If we had to go to the swimming pool for an activity I was always so ashamed.

I would change in the toilet so none of the other kids would see me, but they were onto me. I would get teased for not changing with everyone else.

Skinny girls didn't need to change in the toilet. They changed in the open space. Out and proud! (That was what I thought anyway.)

I would go home at night after one of these days and eat something.

That made me feel better. Momentarily.

Going to someone's house for a sleepover was embarrassing too.

At some point, I would have to change my clothing! I couldn't exactly turn up in my PJs and leave the same way.

They were bound to see *that* roll of fat. Agghhhh.

Going to a party was no fun either.

I felt like everyone would only enjoy talking to the *skinny* girls.

'No boy likes a chubby girl' I would say to myself.

When I *did* go to a party, I felt people would talk to me for a second, just because they *had* to, but they wanted to be talking to the *skinny* girls.

I wasn't being paranoid. This projection actually came true.

They would literally turn their backs and talk to the *skinny* girls.

Looking back, they probably stopped talking to me because I was giving off such a bad paranoid vibe! Not because I had a few extra kgs on my bones.

I didn't know why anyone wanted to talk to me. I wasn't
beautiful enough.
I was so obsessed with *skinny and fat* I couldn't enjoy
myself.
Everything, always, came back to this.

I had ZERO confidence in myself.
Doing any activity at school was embarrassing so I
missed out.
I missed out on being in life and experiencing things
with friends because I was embarrassed of myself.
I thought everyone would be looking at my wobbles. I
had this fixation with being perfect and if I was not
perfect, that meant I would not live life.

At 14, I had started High School and my weight had
gone up and down by 10kgs or so, every year or two.
I participated in sport through High School and was not
bad at running, swimming and netball.
I still had the same paranoia in tow, but it was a little
harder (than Primary School) to get out of an entire
subject, so I participated.

When I was 16, I went to a doctor who specialised in
weight loss.
One of my mum's friends had great success with this
guy, so when I heard about him I begged my parents to
take me along.
I was told to eat bran in the morning with stewed apples
and one orange. One salad roll for lunch with no butter
or cheese and one piece of chicken and a zucchini for
dinner.
I lost weight and looked pretty ok.
I looked 'normal'.
This made me feel OK, but when I stopped *this*

completely unsustainable diet, the weight came back again.
I had formed no great habits or learned <u>anything</u>.
I was simply put on a restricted diet for a period.

When I was 18, I heard about a wonder pill from a girl I had worked with.
I went to the doctor and was prescribed a diet pill.
I looked *so good* after taking this that I could go to nightclubs with my girlfriends and wear hotpants.
I looked damn fine. For about three months.
In the following three months after stopping this pill, I gained practically double what I had lost.
But you will hear all about this little *wonder pill* later…

That high-level summary gives you a little insight into what happened, but how did it make me feel?
Every single day I was tormented by looking in the mirror, traumatised by what I was meant to be.
How I was meant to look.
It ruined my confidence, my self-worth and set me on the path of losing who I was, all in the effort to be something else.
It has made me believe I was less than great in everything I did because I wasn't doing it *skinny*.

As I got into my 20s, everything I talked about previously was still prevalent, just on a larger scale.
Once, my friends put together a beach volleyball team. I joined with them because I was mature enough to get over my fears, but I was the weakest link in the team.
All my girlfriends had been playing sport and participating in things for the last 10 years, and I had only limited experience and zero confidence.
Because of this, I didn't last long. I always felt I was

letting the team down, so I quit.
This is just one example, but this was how my life
panned out.
Participating in as little as possible to prevent
embarrassment.

My twenties is where I mastered the f@!& out of being
a serial dieter.
Oh, boy, did I give it a red hot go!
Even when I was not on a diet I was on a diet.
Every pill, every shake, every weird Internet diet was
experienced.
I was older and I had my own money; this meant I could
try everything that crossed my path.
I even made some of my own diets up.
Yep, you heard it!
I was like a Subway Sandwich Artist... but for diets.
One I recall included *breakfast rice (a special recipe
actually tasty - I may put it in a cookbook one day for
shits and giggles)*, and vegetable soup for the rest of the
day. I thought I was amazing for coming up with these
diets which would make me shed the kgs.
I thought I had found the golden ticket.
Every time.
This was the one.
And every single time, the weight came crawling back
when the willpower to eat one food group disappeared
and my body realised it needed more nourishment than
just veggie soup.

My weight affected my job searching.
I always felt I would not be considered due to not being
hot enough in a pencil skirt; meaning I could not get a
job in an office.
I believed that my appearance was everything.

I believed I had to look <u>great</u> in business attire to even bother looking for a job.

This was not vanity. It was a genuine belief I could not do something because I couldn't wear the skirt. I had tied my entire self-worth and love to being, you guessed it, *skinny*.

I went bungee jumping with friends and was mortified when the bungee company had to weigh me.

Had I known that was a requirement of this activity, I would likely have made up some excuse about fearing heights.

How terrifying! My friends would see I weighed 20kg more than them. AND, they wrote your weight in black marker on your hand! How rude!

That day, my *skinny* friend was petrified of heights and struggled to jump and I was petrified of the black marker.

Then there was clothing.

My wardrobe changed so often because I would fluctuate so much.

I would buy ugly fat clothes, then give them away when I lost weight.

I would then buy clothing that made me feel like <u>me</u> when I was thinner.

I never had *that* awesome pair of jeans I kept for years.

I was lucky to fit into jeans for three months before the weight crawled back on again.

Clothing was not where this ended.

Constantly buying a new nail polish, skin care, hair appliances, handbags…or whatever would make me feel better for being overweight.

The money and time wasted were insane; all on things I felt would make me beautiful in the absence of being thin.

WHAT WAS THE IMPACT?

Many people would think what I am about to say is silly, exaggerated and not the norm.
I beg to differ.
I know I am not special.
I am not here writing this because I believe I am some weirdo who no other person can relate to.
Quite the opposite.
What I know to be true is there are many other women and men out there who feel exactly as I do, but mostly, they don't say it.
I didn't want to talk about it for the longest time either.
It is embarrassing. I get it.

Many people would not understand that when you see someone who has perhaps a few extra kilos on them, there is often something so much more going on in their heart and head when it comes to what they look like.

When you have disordered eating, it is strongly tied to how you feel about your body. And when you feel a certain way about your body, you rarely want to show said body.
You think there is something wrong with it.
You think it is the only thing that matters.
You think it doesn't look as it should. And if it isn't how it should be, you are embarrassed to show it.

It is hard to live life without your body in tow, so you opt out of life… well, parts of it anyway.

In my time, there have been many things I didn't do, because I felt my body was not right for the occasion.

Here are some:

- Go out with friends
- Apply for a job I loved doing
- Do a course I wanted to do – because only hot, thin people did *that* course
- Continue being a fitness instructor (because I wasn't skinny enough)
- Continue being a Food Coach (because my body was not a reflection on my eating so how on earth could I continue this)
- Be confident in front of men (and often women)
- Participate in group sports
- Participate in <u>active</u> activities at work (work and lycra do not mix)
- Go bungee jumping at a work function (I knew they would have to weigh me, that had happened before and NO THANK YOU – and what if I had to wear a wetsuit and it didn't fit??)
- Get in the pool at a friend's place
- Go to the beach with friends
- Walk around certain towns
- Talk to people at parties
- Leave the house
- Run

  And much more… I have blocked it all out of my mind. :)

Not doing the above-mentioned activities has shaped my life differently.

I feel like I have missed out on doing things, however, I also feel like at the time, there was no option.

I was scared for no reason because many of the above situations would have been fun, rewarding and most likely, not embarrassing.

We have ideas in our head about what 'good' looks like in our society. But what if for a second, I decided, I will love and accept myself because I feel good?

What if I could never change? What if this is who I was and I had to be happy with what is?

I am who I am right now.

I cannot change what I look like but I can change how I respond to situations.

I can say yes more. I can wear clothing that makes me feel comfortable and do *the thing*. Whatever that thing is.

I can choose to not miss out, and then while I am not missing out, I am forgetting about what I look like and I am participating in life.

And the more you are participating in life, the more you heal.

And when you heal, you no longer have an eating disorder in the front seat of your life. There is no room for it.

You are so busy *doing stuff* there is no room for anything else.

And when there is no room for anything else, you are leading the life you always wanted, doing *all the things*, talking to *all the people*.

And if you are leading this life, isn't that all you need?

<u>That</u> is when you realise that you can do *life* with that extra 10kg on. And the weight need not be <u>gone</u> before you start living life. Losing 10, 20 or 30kg is not the gateway to happiness you have been waiting to 'jimmy' open.
It is all in your head, it is all your choice. You can start participating today, with or without the 10kg hugging your thighs.

Here are a few things I did to help me start living:

- Bought myself a few nice pieces of clothing!
- Faked it till I made it! If you at least have a few items of clothing that make you feel like you, you can participate in life comfortably.
- I had to not care. It did not serve me to hide.
- I danced the Zorba in my bathers with a boat full of people watching me whilst travelling the Greek islands. I cannot stand being the center of attention, so this was a real feat for me.

Say Yes.
Push through the feeling that wants to say no. Just start participating more.
The funny thing is when you participate in the first few activities you would have normally said 'no' to, you realise the world does not implode and nobody is pointing and laughing at you, you realise it isn't that bad and you can then participate
more and more.
A journey of a thousand miles begins with just one step. Once you try one thing, you will gain the confidence to do another, and another.

For most of us, confidence is built. Some of us are not lucky enough to be born with it. So, we just need to take one step at a time.

Over the years I have said 'no' to life.
'No' to things that would make me happy; all because of my body.
Now I say 'No More' to saying no.

And for those of you wondering if I am still scared sometimes? Maybe for a millisecond, but it disappears quickly once I dive right in.

It's never as bad as you think it will be.

MY LIFE LESSONS from THE BEGINNING:

- Never tell a child they are fat.
There are so many other ways you could help them if they don't seem healthy. Telling them they are fat is not one of them.
- Never compare children to anyone else.
They are all unique and beautiful little humans in their own way.
- People mean no harm when they say you are fat. They just don't know any better.
- Always encourage others to be healthy because it feels good.
Encourage playful movement.
- My parents are seriously the best parents in the world. #Blessed
- All doctors and professionals are not suited to all people.
Find the ones that suit you best and align with your values.
- There is no such thing as a naughty food. Making something naughty attaches guilt.
- Never put a child on a diet. Teach them how to eat properly to start with.
- You need not look good in a pencil skirt to have a good career.
- I will never say no to anything because of the way I look.

Chapter 3 – A Life of Diets

Just to be clear, AGAIN, I am not a dietitian.
But as far as I know Google, isn't one either and she is allowed to tell the world what a diet is…
So, let's start with Google's dictionary definition.

Diet:
noun
1.
the kinds of food that a person, animal, or community habitually eats.
"a vegetarian diet"

2.
a special course of food to which a person restricts themselves, either to lose weight or for medical reasons.
"I'm **going on a diet**"

I have a very strong opinion on the above two definitions.
Description 1. Is what everyone should have.
Description 2. Should be reserved for medical reasons.

WHAT IS A DIET?

So many people use description 2 (above), me included, for reasons other than medical, and sometimes, the act of dieting itself turns into a medical emergency when people create life-threatening eating disorders or diseases.

Dieting for weight loss when not required for medical reasons should be taught at schools as something that can be **as life-threatening and bad for your health as**

smoking or drugs. But hey… I am clearly a little passionate about that.

I feel kids should be taught about all the great things real food and moving well does to their body. They should not be separated from the thinner kids and be made to exercise more (fat-shamed and embarrassed) which is what I heard the government were thinking of doing this week on the news.

You may remember earlier, I mentioned that even when I wasn't on a diet, I was on a diet.
Let me elaborate on this one a little.

There were times, that I was definitely on a diet. It was very clear.
I would follow a regime prescribed by a person, book or course I was taking. The times in between, I would still be in the diet mentality. Restricting, feeling guilt and emotionally tormenting myself for not having stuck to the previous diet a little longer.

I tried the same diets more than once, but diets rarely worked as well the second time.
I think it's because I was scarred by the previous experience.
Trying a new one held new hope.
Maybe *this* was the one I could stick to forever?

When I tried to do the math on *my* dieting over the years I came up with a very conservative $5000 spend per year.
All because I didn't know how to eat on my own?

This includes all the things I did and purchased to make me feel beautiful or thin.

A caveman could get from A-B and figure out how to eat without an app or doctor telling them how. Meanwhile, I was beating myself up because I couldn't figure out something as simple as eating on my own. It made no sense. How had we as humans forgotten how to manage one of the most basic primal instincts?

Think about it.
Do you know how many diets there are?
Do you know how many weight loss devices, memberships, pills, courses, there are?
The thing is, I've been a sucker.
And I have tried a good chunk of them.

SOMETIMES IT'S A DIET IN DISGUISE

Sometimes, I have thought I wasn't on a diet, but it had been a diet in disguise.

Like when I purchased a Fitness Tracker.
I, like many others, purchased a fitness tracker, believing it would make me fit(and thin).

What I did find is that after a week, I knew I had to walk for 45 minutes a day, plus my normal incidental walking to reach my 10,000 steps.
So why did I need a device after I had learned this?

That, tied into calorie tracking and the need to measure and judge myself based on a few numbers on a screen, became another diet.

I am sure there is a time and a place for fitness trackers;
perhaps for athletes? But for someone like me, who just
wants to be healthy and fit, the measuring is
unnecessary.
A fitness tracker was not inspirational once the novelty
faded.
Inspirational was finding movement I loved to do and
having the nous to alter this often enough to keep me
feeling good, happy and motivated.

I have found that health is more sustainable and natural
when done intuitively to feel good, rather than judging
myself by looking at a number on a screen.
Nine thousand steps in a day will not make me a failure.

Even when I wasn't dieting I was thinking about food.
Not in a daydreamy sort of way… more like a paranoia
and unhealthy obsession with it.
If someone offered me something I would calculate
calories in my mind, analyse the ingredients and wonder
if that would later cause some binges.
My friend coined me 'the packet princess'. She did not
understand that I would prefer eating foods from a
packet because they had a nutrition panel on them that
would help me record my calories.
I think she just thought I didn't like eating fresh food.

There was even a time where I thought I was healthy
and into 'clean eating' but that was just another version
of an unhealthy obsession with only good foods. I gave
myself no flexibility.
Even if I wasn't tracking calories, mentally I was
categorising foods as good and bad and would punish
myself for not sticking to the list diligently.

There is a name for this. Orthorexia is when you are obsessed with being healthy and only eating foods that are healthy. For me, it was just another diet in disguise that would end in a pile of mess.

WHAT'S SO WRONG WITH DIETS ANYWAY?

I have found that diets have never worked.
I thought a diet 'working' was that I would complete the 'X' weeks required to lose the weight and I would be done.
And then, I would never have to go on a diet again.
I thought that once I was *skinny*, I would be healed. I knew I would have to maintain health, (and I wanted to) but I thought it would be easier if I was skinny.

That was never the case.
There are no 'diets' that work <u>in my 'book'</u>. *Having* a good diet differs greatly from being on a diet.

There is something very wrong with doing something temporarily and expecting long lasting results.
Especially with health.
I feel really dumb as I am writing this, having not realised it sooner.

In my defense, I think deep down I knew a diet was not going to work forever, but I was desperate.
I would've had an event to go to and I just couldn't wait.
I needed to be thin in two months, so off I went on the diet train again.

Speaking of desperate, I did mention at the start of the book I was going to be 100% transparent with everything I did. Below, I am going to share with you a few of the diets I tried in my most desperate times.

1. Doctor-Prescribed Diet Pills - initially when 18 years old

Are you familiar with the commercial on Australian TV which depicts a woman being weighed in a doctor's surgery?

It is the commercial where the doctor sees the patient has lost 2 kg, then suddenly starts dancing around the surgery screaming and congratulating the patient?

This is not some great program for you to follow, simply a quick-fix pill.

The pill I took makes your heart race like mad, and you cannot sleep when you take it.

You lay awake in bed feeling the bones in your hips and how empty your stomach feels.

You can barely eat and you drink so much you are constantly on the toilet.

You don't think about food at all and your mouth is so dry you look like there is something wrong with you.

I am sure there is a good amount of amphetamines in this tablet too. Hence the no sleep. Like speed.

You lose crap loads of weight and it can send you crazy. Like loopy. It did that to me.

You also eat so little it is difficult to go to the loo for number 2's. But being obsessed with losing weight, I also took laxatives to help this process along.

After a while, it stops working and everything comes crashing down.

There are two different doses, so as it stops being effective, the doctor puts you on a higher dose.

Once you <u>stop</u> taking it, you become tired.
I am talking, I couldn't get out of bed, literally couldn't get up, needed to sleep for three days straight.
It makes sense to be so tired if you haven't had a good sleep for two months.
THEN, you wake up and eat everything.
You become so freaking hungry that you eat it ALL.
All the time. That weight you just lost is back **x 2** in a matter of weeks.

"Thank you, medical system for providing me with a ridiculous drug that is not doing anything positive for my health AT ALL. Yeah, my BMI was in the healthy weight range for two weeks. But now my eating disorder is even worse, and I feel even more shit about myself than ever before."

The doctor will tell you this is safe and OK. They will tell you with a balanced healthy diet and exercise it will help you form good habits but that is just not true. I have seen this happen to friends too. I had one friend completely lose her marbles.

2. Becoming Vegetarian
I was a teen when I did this, and outwardly I did it for 'moral' reasons but honestly, I thought becoming a vegetarian would help me lose weight. So, I tried this for about a year till I walked past a Kebab shop and smelt that luscious lamb and realised I really needed some of that in my belly.
This put a stop to that little experiment.
To this day, I am still not a big red meat eater. But I don't think I ever want to say *never*.
I eat red meat occasionally.

3. The Low GI diet

Because I struggle to do things in halves, once I read the 'low GI diet', I needed to ONLY eat foods that were going to burn slowly in my system.

That was the answer!

If I only ate foods that burnt slowly, then I would be hungry less often and naturally lose this weight.

Easy Peas-y.

The only problem is you are restricting a whole lot of food if you only eat low GI foods.

4. Pharmacy Shakes

I have tried all the brands at various stages of my life. They are revolting and consuming these are a completely unsustainable way of life. Water and powder are not food.

5. The Blood Type Diet

Like the GI diet, I read a book about eating right for your blood type and decided I was only going to eat foods that were on my blood type list. Again, not a sustainable way to live. There are some good concepts in there which I agree with (like each body type is not suited to all foods) but I have found trial and error to be more effective in finding what suits my body and makes me feel good.

6. Various Dietitians

I have visited dietitians who have prescribed a specific diet, but on two separate occasions, I was prescribed shakes. I didn't feel that was how to go when I was trying to figure out how to eat normally.

7. Various Naturopaths
Like my experience with dietitians, restricted programs, and prescribing shakes didn't really set me up for long-term success.

8. Garcinea Cambogia Tablets
This was the latest fad in health food stores for a while. Designed to burn fat with a healthy diet. The healthy diet alone would have done the trick.

9. The Cambridge Diet
Another version of shakes but made out to be a little more scientific than the generic pharmacy style products.

10. HCG Diet
I can't decide whether this was the worst diet I have ever been on or not. It is up there! I won't spoil the surprise as I delve into this one a little later.

Remember these are just a few… there would surely be 100's of diets and dollars spent that my brain simply can't go back that far to list them all.

Also, it may not be fair of me to say these ALL don't work.
They may work for you.

And, it may not be fair to say that <u>every inventor</u> of a new diet is doing it with the intention of making money alone.
I am sure they want you to succeed.
I am sure they want lots of people to succeed so they can help <u>many people,</u> and I am also sure that many may have big hearts and they would love to help the world.

For me, anything but inserting a new habit I love and want to do is not the way I like to roll these days. I don't subscribe to challenges, short-term programs, or anything with an expiry date.

WHO IS TO BLAME?

It is hard to pinpoint the starting line.
What came first the chicken or the egg?

We can look at the diet industry and blame them, we can look at the education system, we can look at each other. We are all to blame, but revolution does not come from blame.

You must always do your best until you know better.

Over the years, in my journey of healing, I have written things about diet companies and industries doing wrong by us.
About experts not really caring about our health. About ways things could be better, but how is that helpful?
I can't take the whole diet industry and remove it from earth.
There was originally going to be an entire chapter about it... but what's the point of looking backward when I want to go forward?

It would also be easy to blame people in your life for contributing to your failures too, but I really believe we are predestined to live a certain life.
YES, we create and shape our own lives, but I think I was meant to learn all I have learned to help inspire change in others, so they don't have to suffer.

I also believe that you should use what happens to you for *good not evil*.

There is no point in pointing a finger at the boyfriend who dumped you. Or the kid in the schoolyard who called you fat. Or the relative who thought they were doing right by you. I can't even blame the doctor who came to my school when I was seven who kicked off this diet merry-go-round. Everyone was just doing the best they could at the time with the knowledge and experience they had.

It is very rare that someone has done something to you with intention of hurting you.

I don't have the stats on that, but I am sure less than .1% of the time you are hurt is intentional, and the rest of the time you are bearing the brunt of misunderstanding or somebody not educated on a topic as you are.

I have decided blame is <u>not</u> the way forward.
I know better now, so I am doing better.

I have educated myself and hopefully inspire change.

I've found that spending more time and energy on the 'get-better-game' gave me a much better result than focusing on the 'blame-game'.

DIETS FOR EVENTS

I am giving this its own heading because I have realised that most of the time I've spent dieting was *for* something.

An event is not necessarily something that comes with an invitation.

It could have been for something obvious, like a party or a holiday. But, often 'events' were less obvious things. Like to impress a guy, or to start the new year, or because I had a new job, or because I wanted to wear a certain size or play a certain sport, or because I was turning a certain age.

Everything in my life was an 'event' I needed to get thin for.

Life was constantly on hold because I was waiting to get thin first. And when it wasn't on hold, it was tainted by the feeling of failure as I hadn't gotten to where I needed to be, thin.

Even when I was thinner I wasn't thin enough.

When I decided to quit diets, I remember thinking, what am I going to do about this person's wedding? Or that holiday? Or people at work?

Will they all think I am a lesser person because I am not thin?

Will I look like a failure? Or like I have let myself go? Or will they be thinking I should go on a diet (not realising that's what got me into this mess)?

There is such a massive culture of praising someone who is dieting and getting thin. "Well done, for *temporarily* starving yourself and embarking on an unsustainable way of life. You look great"

Nobody could see the work I was doing inside. There was no outward appearance of success. Quite the opposite.

In a culture where thin is better, I almost felt like I had to apologise for my weight gain when I quit dieting.

Like I wanted to tell people, "I am healing, a long-term issue, you just can't see it yet, this is temporary"

I had to come to terms with how I would best deal with events.
Every event was a trigger to diet. So, everything in my life was going to try and reel me back into that diet merry-go-round. This was one of the most challenging things.

I had to think, 'what was more important'?
Being embarrassed at an event for not looking 'my best'? Or embarking on a long-term healing journey that would make me healthy forever?

You can guess what I chose.
Because I had become a Lion. :)

WORKING FOR A HEALTH FOOD COMPANY

After nine years of working in software and IT, I decided I needed a career change and dove into an industry really close to my heart. Health. Specifically, Health Food.

I got what at the time felt like the best job, working for a health food distributor.
I was going to speak with customers all day about great healthy products and work with like-minded people, learning about the latest trends in health.

Like with anything new, the start was exciting. I would use a good chunk of my salary purchasing the latest products and super foods to add to my repertoire(to help create my own diets at home).

It was clearly an integral part of my journey, as this two year stint highlighted, in BIG BOLD FLURO PINK, that the health food industry was just another gravy train, filling consumers with hope for health.

Being submerged in the superfluous amounts of products that would be released every month, all with the tag 'super food' on them, made me question and research all of these products.
Often, I would find that the protein in these 'high protein' products was <u>nothing</u> compared to a boiled egg. Or often I found that the nutrients in a super powder would be of equal value to an apple.
It really made me question not only diets but all the fad products that people (like me) were suckered into purchasing, all in the name of health.

Was a 'super powder' that necessary when I was filling my plate with veggies? Was the superfood seed mix necessary, when I could continue to buy pumpkin seeds from the local store?

I am grateful for my time in the industry as it really highlighted everything that <u>was not</u> a version of healthy I was striving for.

Good whole foods, like Grandma used to have, were all I needed. Not the powdered version of a salad.

MY LIFE LESSONS from A LIFE OF DIETS:

- I have a diet, I'm not on one.
- If you feel guilty about what you are eating, you may
  be on a diet
- I don't need pedometers and fitness trackers to help
  me get fit
- Diets have not taught me to eat.

They have taught me I am a failure for not being able to stick to them forever.

- There is nobody to blame but the diet itself.
- I do not have to be skinny to go to a friend's wedding.
- Health food is not necessarily healthy.
- Eat an apple.

Chapter 4 – The Catalyst

THE LEAD UP TO DECIDING TO QUIT DIETS

One does not just decide to quit diets.
A lot needs to happen to get you to that point in your
life. Especially when it is something that has consumed
you for so long.
I suppose if you do something for a few months, or a
couple of years, quitting it may not be as hard?
I guess it would depend on what you were trying to
quit!?

I think the main problem with quitting something that is
causing you pain is figuring out that it is the thing that
is, in fact, causing the pain!

I don't think if you'd asked me 10 years ago, if I thought
dieting was my issue, I would have understood.
I would have been blindsided by your suggestion.

Ten years ago, I thought I had no willpower. Or I was
just not meant to be thinner or healthy.
I thought I was failing the diets. I didn't realise the diets
were failing me.
I just thought that was how I was.
I kept looking at relatives who were mainly overweight
and thinking it must have had something to do with my
genes which I do understand play a part. However, I
think when it comes to good health, nature, and nurture
combined play a part in most cases.

I feel confident in guessing that there may be some
extreme cases where a person has no say in their health.
Perhaps where a condition is passed on from family, of
they have an illness or disease.

But in most cases, we can get ourselves healthy with proper care of our mind, body, and soul. Using whichever means we like. We are spoiled for choice. :)

Earlier in the book, I touched on a few of the diets that took center stage over the years. As I said, there had been too many to remember or count. Right here is where I will share with you exactly what tipped me over the edge and funnily enough, a diet I embarked on when I was 36 was the catalyst in me making the decision to finally quit. Forever.
I guess that is not uncommon.
You hear of drug addicts or alcoholics having that one, last, life-changing experience that makes them run for the hills and turn their life around.

It kinda played out like that.
And I guess, like a drug addict, with diets and food being my addiction, I had always dreamed of quitting. But I just couldn't.
Diets were so exciting. Being on a diet was when I didn't feel like a failure. I was achieving something, and I was looking better.
Having weigh-ins, feeling your flat tummy, all the attention, the momentary self-confidence in a life of feeling never quite good enough.
The self-acceptance of dropping a dress size, feeling like I had finally made it. I was a worthy human because I was wearing a size 10.
From never being enough, I was now complete.

But all the while, simultaneously, as this 'high' of losing weight was occurring, I was also wishing I would never have to do this again. Always wishing this was the last one. I just wanted to be a normal person. I didn't at the time understand that the diets themselves were making me unhealthy. I thought they were healthy, and I was 'bad' for not being able to sustain the diet way of life.

Don't get me wrong, I was not completely stupid. I did understand a life of moderation was the way to go (somewhere deep down), but moderation doesn't drop 10 kilos in 4 weeks.
The plan was almost always to 'do the diet' for 4-12 weeks (depending on what plan I was being prescribed and how much weight I 'needed' to lose) and then move to a life of moderation.

There were two problems with this plan;

1) It is rare that a diet focuses on after the diet.
Lots of them include some sort of obligatory maintenance plan at the back of the book, but that part is not what sells the diet. It's an afterthought.
It should be the main part.
That itself should be the diet. But that's not as sexy as dropping weight in lightning speed, is it?
Would the companies get buy-in if the ad told you to expect 10kg weight loss in two years?
Doubtful.

2) Most diets focus on massive calorie restriction or food group restriction. Even foods you don't normally like to eat enter your fantasies when you may not eat them.
So, when the blessed 'diet' is over and you reach that weight or start feeling good about yourself the diet is done!

And gradually you start eating all the things you missed out on.

And the weight piles back on.

The act of restriction just makes you want the food that much more when the diet is done. That doesn't set you up for a good maintenance plan.

On the day I quit diets, I was elbow-deep in the diet of my life.

It was next-level stupid, dangerous and unnecessary. But I didn't think that at the time.

I was desperate.

Remember earlier I spoke about the importance *events* had played in my dieting?

Well, *he* had just put a ring on it, and this opened the floodgates for a plethora of emotions and ridiculous thoughts.

Here are some:

1. I wanted to be a beautiful bride (that's an obvious one)

2. I wanted to start our new life as husband and wife thin, and then never go on a diet again (I sort of achieved this, but I wouldn't exactly call it a success, you will hear about that soon).

3. My Hubby's ex-wife was larger and I didn't want him to have another large wife.

4. I didn't want my Hubby's family to feel sorry for him marrying someone who wasn't thin (WTF, seriously WTF). By the way, I was fairly *normal* in size for the 4 years we were together prior to the wedding.

So, with that ridiculous visual in your mind I started some at home do it yourself diets.

Feeling the pressure of the date creeping closer and closer, I got desperate when the weight wasn't moving as rapidly as I wanted.

I went to the GP after seeing a commercial on TV advertising how 'your local GP can help you lose weight'. I thought that sounded like a great idea! Having someone to check-in with and guide me with their professional opinion sounded just the ticket!

When I started talking to the doctor, after mentioning the commercial, I just knew this was not going to be the solution I was looking for. He told me the commercial was referring to diet pills. Remember that terrible drug that had caused me so much pain 18 years earlier? Yeah, that stuff.

I went home, desperate to find something else. I did some research and stumbled across what seemed to be the best diet in the world. 'How had I not found this one before?' I thought to myself.

This was it! I could do this diet forever!!!

Enter HCG.

The HCG Diet is sold well.

For a diet aficionado like myself, who likes to be sold on the facts, stats, and prestige of a ground-breaking diet, this one certainly did the trick.

I read the book in a night and decided I needed to get started ASAP!

This book had everything I needed to convince me this was not a diet. It was *different*.
It's not even called a diet. It's technically called The HCG Protocol.

The gist of this diet is:
Start taking hormone drops from a pregnant woman (under your tongue), designed to suppress appetite, amongst other things.
For the first three days you 'load' - this means you need to eat everything you possibly can that is <u>fatty</u>.
All the junk food.
All the butter you can fit in.
Then move to a diet of 600 calories for 21 days. (Where you starve yourself and fantasise about food for three weeks.)
Finally, you stop taking the hormones, about 7kg lighter.

You are meant to go on this diet, wait a month and then do it again. Each time losing about 7 kg (results vary).

When I started this diet, I thought to myself, 'Oh this is perfect, I can manage 21 days, once a year, to shed anything I may have gained throughout the year.' I thought it was the perfect way to maintain my weight. A small-time investment once a year. Easy.

What nobody prepared me for was the feeling inside when the hormones stopped.
I was so hungry I couldn't even function or think straight. I just needed to eat.
In the days after the hormones stop, you are still meant to maintain a 600-calorie diet. You are warned that you can put all the weight back on if you don't.

There was no way on earth I was able to do this! I was ravenous and exhausted.
Not to mention weak!
You are not allowed to exercise while on the HCG protocol (600 calories barely give you enough energy to do the basics in life) so I had lost muscle mass and was unfit.

From being a healthy woman with a few extra kilos on her, who had just completed a half marathon, I went to a weak, ravenous, binge eater who wanted to eat everything in sight.

I put all the weight back on in about 4 days.

This terrified me and I started having flashbacks to 18 years earlier at how fast I dropped the weight when I took prescribed tablets from the doctor (Remember the diet pills?).

I was desperate. I had a plan. But I had little time up my sleeve now.

I went back to the original doctor, hanging my head in shame and asked for the diet pills.
I must tell you, this went against every grain in my body. Every moral standard. Against Everything I knew was right.
Internally I knew I was doing the wrong thing.
I mean these tablets are not only bad because of the diet yo-yo they send you on, they have serious side effects like heart problems, depression and worse.
I didn't want to take them, but the need to be skinny FAR outweighed anything else.

I wasn't allowed to do the HCG protocol for another month, so I thought if I could take the tablets for a month, lose the weight (which I had just lost and put back on again), I would be in a better place and could do another round of HCG.

Good plan, right?? I'm full of bright ideas!?!

The next four months in the lead up to the wedding were a series of back to back HCG sessions with diet pills in between to ensure the weight was not put back on for the wedding. Brilliant.

REALISING I NEVER WANTED TO DIET AGAIN

Somewhere during the most dangerous, unhealthy, idiotic thing I have ever done, came clarity.

I hated what I was doing but could not see a way out until the wedding was over.
Morally, I was resolute. I would never diet, EVER again. I would have my beautiful wedding day and then move to a life of moderation.
In my quest for normality, in true Kelly fashion, I googled the crap out of 'how to eat normally', 'how do you eat in moderation?', 'how do normal people eat?'.
I stumbled across lots of sites and ideas that inspired me to make a change.
One favourite was by two health professionals from Melbourne who had created a Facebook page called 'The Moderation Movement'.
They posted messages and quotes that were instrumental

in cementing the ideas that were already burning within me.

From a food perspective, this did the trick, but for me, there was more to it than simply making a choice to 'eat like a normal person'.

A massive mindset change needed to happen. I needed to work on *why* I was dieting for all these years, and *why* I no longer should.
The need for self-care and learning to properly love myself had to come first.

I just couldn't live like this anymore.
The idea of being on and off diets, loving and hating myself, sounded like the most pathetic roller-coaster ride at Disneyland.

After all that's said and done, if you can be proud of your actions and what you have created, you are OK.
If you can look at your life and say you have done your best, then there is not much more you could wish for.
Dieting was not me at my best. It was me hating myself.
I was not caring for myself. I was hurting myself.
For years.

I decided I was going to quit, and never weigh myself again… but I still had a couple of months till the wedding, so I wasn't going to stop yet.

WAS QUITTING DIETS EASY?

The act of quitting diets itself was easy.
Unlike the addiction of alcoholism, you are quitting a
life of restriction and are all of a sudden free to do what
you like.

There is a freedom in quitting dieting. You don't feel
like you are missing out on something like alcoholism.
Quite the opposite.
You have a new menu of things to choose from that had
for so long been rarely seen as acceptable in your eyes.

I rewarded myself for 30+ years of restriction and
torture by eating everything in moderation.
EVERYTHING.

Yes, I had read a few quotes and inspirational books
popped into my life to help me decide to quit, but
looking back, I didn't know how to do this.

What was moderation?
And after 30+ years of restriction, what did I even like?
What was my favourite food?
What did I NOT like?
I had no idea how to eat like a normal person.
I thought I did, but it didn't come naturally.

I went to the other extreme.

I felt like I *deserved* to not have to worry about food.
I felt like I was being kind to myself by not having to
think twice about a portion size.
My body was saying *'lady, you have tortured me for*

30+ years and now I am going to do whatever the hell I like and I am going to hold onto every little thing you put into me with all my might'.

I felt like it was *my right* to just have a break from caring about food for a few months.

I craved foods I was never allowed to eat and allowed myself to eat them. Sometimes even two. Three even.

It felt so good to start with, just being free.

Then my clothes stopped fitting.

At that point, I wasn't sure what to do.

I thought to myself, '*I will stop gaining weight once my body gets this out of its system.*'

I thought the cravings would level-out once I had given my body the freedom to eat what it wanted.

'Once I give myself permission to eat anything my body craves and stop depriving myself, I won't desire these things anymore' is what I thought.

About six months in, I was up two dress sizes and still resolute that I would find a healthy way of weight maintenance on my own.

I wasn't sure how, but I was confident it would happen naturally.

Twelve months in I was the largest I had ever been and decided to weigh myself.

I needed to know the number.

Even though weighing myself was going against everything I had just learned. Even though I knew I was not a number, I just needed to know.

I had gained 25 kilos.

My body had aches and pains all over.

My once fit body felt flabby, and for the first time ever I had cellulite.

Quitting diets was easy…
My lack of preparation and forethought of how massive that would be, after years of dieting was not.

If I knew then what I know now, the next three years would not have been nearly as hard.
But I guess that would mean I wouldn't have been able to share my successes and mistakes with you here;
Which will hopefully help you in your journey.
I will share more on this soon!

WHAT IS A BINGE?

When you realise you may have an actual issue, shit gets real.

I will never forget when I realised my binging and food addiction was an issue, a real thing.
It took me by surprise. Kinda like a bowling ball to the gut surprise, not your hubby taking you to Tiffany's *to choose the biggest diamond* kind of surprise.

A binge is different things for different people and I can only tell you what it was for me.

All my life I just thought I was just naughty or a piggy when I came in and out of diets and binged on the foods I had deprived myself of.
It took me a while to realise that something was

happening on a very emotional and chemical level. And it wasn't until that realisation was I able to fix it.

What a binge was for me:

Being a mega-healthy eater all my life, junk food had a purpose. I didn't like it. I am THAT girl that loves broccoli and brussel sprouts. Grilled chicken excites me. 'Avo' and poached eggs are yummy.
Salad, well in my opinion, you DO win friends with salad.
I don't try to eat healthy. I just love healthy food (Good job, Mum).

A binge was nothing to do with the food. The food was a vehicle. A chemical to mask the pain. A tool to deal with the anxiety and as it turns out, it was a plain addiction.

There were so many times over the years I binged, emotionally ate or overate.

Here are some of those times:

- When I was put on a diet by the family doctor at seven years old. I would hide to eat.
- When I was bored and had nothing to do; I was an only child and it was a way to pass time.
- When my parents divorced and I had to stay at home while they were at work sometimes. I again was lonely. TV and a snack(s)were my company.
- When people would tease me.
- When the self-loathing was so bad only drinking would take it away. Followed by late night gorges.

- When I was so lonely that I dated a guy that was just not right. And on the way home from his place, I would eat, eat, eat…
- When I was alone in another country, there was nothing else to comfort me.
- When I would diet several times a year, and the derivative of this would be, of course, binge eating.
- When I did not feel good enough.
- When I got married and starved myself, and again could not stop eating after the starving myself was over.
- When I would feel anxious about not getting everything done that needed to get done.
- When I was finally addicted to the process of dieting and certain foods and for no reason, just couldn't stop. It had become a habit.

A binge episode would look different each time. Sometimes it would be standing in the kitchen and going from cupboard to fridge eating everything. Sometimes I would order food. Sometimes I would stop and buy three or 4 bits of junk food. Sometimes I would do that several times a day.

Why did I do it?
I still don't know *why* food was the answer. I mean, I wish I could remember what set it off… But after years of studying the reasons, visiting professionals, searching my soul and delving into childhood memories, I believe it's because it started by filling some sort of void, rebelling against what I was being restricted from and in the end, a plain addiction to the sugar. There was a need

to feed my mouth when I should have been feeding my soul.

As I was eating the food I felt calm. It was literally like a drug, calming me down, and as soon as I stopped eating the anxiety would start again; so, I would reach for my next drug of choice in the form of some kind of snack food.

How did I recognise it was a problem?
Well, that answer came from a combination of things.

When I started asking (hinting to) friends about their eating habits and they did not have the same experience, I knew there was something wrong.
I thought everybody had times where they felt so anxious that they would eat everything in the house until they felt sick, – sitting down, then going back for more once that packet was finished. I thought they all would do this until their gut hurt so much they were keeled over in pain. I thought it was normal to break out in pimples, to want to vomit and feel like never getting out of bed.
Well kinda. Deep down I knew that wasn't really the case. I guess I just never wanted to admit there was something wrong.

The other glaringly obvious indicator was the fact that I was miserable, and I did not feel like myself when I was doing this. Remember back to when I said I was a very healthy eater?
Well, these binges were different from my normal eating. There was my normal eating, and then this other thing that happened that involved this other food-like

'stuff' that was more like a drug than a food.
There was my real food and then this druggy gross food.
Two separate things.

I had labeled certain foods as naughty so early on that I
had never given myself permission to eat these foods
even in moderation. It felt like it was only something I
could do secretly.

Other indicators were:

> Depression – because I was not living my true life.
> Helplessness – because I could not see a way out.
> Desperateness – because all I ever wanted was to be
> me.

How did I fix it?
This may not be the easy response you were looking for,
but you guessed it.
I worked damn hard.

I attribute my recovery to work, work and more work.
Worky-workington. Workville. The Work.
All the Work.

I knew my eating disorder was not the end. I would not
live my whole life not living my life.
I was not being me.
You cannot possibly be yourself when you are not
happy.
Life is meant to be lived, with joy and happiness. Not
feeling constantly defeated and out of your skin.

IT TOOK A LONG TIME

I don't want to scare anyone reading this looking for
inspiration.
There is a happily ever after!

When I made the choice to quit diets, I was unprepared.

It wasn't until I was a year in, majorly depressed, with
the realisation I needed some help, did I get a firecracker
up my bottom!

Had I done what I did a year in, on the day I decided to
quit diets, my outlook and journey would have been
very different.

I was not prepared.
I just quit.
Not facing the years of damage, mentally and physically
to my body.
I thought I could do it on my own. I had this idea in my
mind I was sick of spending my money on diets and
things to make me feel better.
My plan was this: I would eat whatever I wanted for a
few months, and then move to a life of moderation.

I hadn't thought of the fact that eating crap food would
lead to an addiction to more crap food. I hadn't thought
that this would be something that was going to be hard
to stop.
I didn't think that this would turn into full-blown daily
binges.
I mean, how could it? I was no longer restricting myself,
so why would I need to?

My loving husband kept telling me I needed to forget
the idea that I would return to my version of a healthy
size in a couple of months.
He was right.

I mean, I had spent over 30 years dieting and being up
and down like a yo-yo.
What if I could spend a year or two or three on proper
healing? And set myself up for a life more balanced?

When you compare a couple of years to a lifetime of
potential dieting, it doesn't seem that long. Especially
when trying to achieve long-term health. Not a number
on a scale.

My mindset had to change. I had to remove all obstacles
from my way.
There was no way I would give up until I had created a
healthy sustainable life of inner peace and balance.
My goals changed from numbers to feelings.

It's amazing how this alone, makes you feel like you
have already succeeded.

In saying this, I feel like I need to add a disclaimer.
Healing will vary for everyone.
We are all at different stages in life with access to
different resources and in need of different help.
Had I been more prepared, I would have achieved what I
felt was 'healed' at least a year prior.
Maybe even two.

Surrounding myself with people who could help me succeed in my goals was key.

And understanding there were many elements at play was important to learn.

I wasn't just 'in bad habits'. I didn't just 'have a bad mindset'. The early dieting habits did not create this alone. There wasn't something chemically wrong with me. I wasn't born hating myself.

There were so many pieces of the puzzle I had to work on and I still have to work on them all.

Intuitive eating alone will not cure me. Daily exercise is not enough. Regular appointments with a psychologist are not the answer alone.

There is really no way to determine what came first. The chicken or the egg? The self-loathing or the diet? The food addiction or the lack of willpower?

I am resolute that everything just happened for a reason and everything just fueled the fire.

MY LIFE LESSONS from THE CATALYST:

- You don't know what you don't know.
Don't beat yourself up over that. Hindsight is a
wonderful thing.
- Diet's give you a similar high to taking a drug.
You feel like you are on top of the world. When the diet
is over so is the high and the weight piles on again. This
is the come down.
- The size on your clothing does not make you a good
    or bad person.
- Self-Acceptance should only come from knowing you
    are trying to be the best
person you can be. Not because of a number on the
scale.
- Restriction is not the same thing as eating everything
    in moderation or
eating intuitively.
- You can be a beautiful bride if you are a beautiful
    person inside.
You need not lose 10kg for the occasion.
- Diet pills and quick fixes are never the answer.
Especially if you feel like it goes against everything you
believe in.
- It's not going to be easy, but it will be worth it!
- If I had my time over, I would have booked a session
    with a specialist or
psychologist the day I decided to quit diets.
- I need not hide foods I eat.

Chapter 5 – Moving and Shaking

WHAT DID ALL THIS MEAN FOR MY HEALTH AND FITNESS?

Weight fluctuation and improper diet affected my body.
I had aches and pains, trouble bending over in yoga class
and reaching places I could normally reach.
All the food restriction had meant there were times I
couldn't exercise the way I was used to or wanted to.

I went from running easily every day to feeling like my
knees were going to explode if I started a light jog.

Unfortunately, exercise and fitness get dragged into
eating disorders. They kinda go hand in hand.
When counting calories, you are balancing numbers,
measuring calories burned and somewhere along the
way you forget what you love and you only have eyes
for the exercises which produce the highest caloric burn.

I suppose you could have an eating disorder without
having an issue with exercise, but this has not been my
experience. I have been super fit over the years, and
super unfit.
Just like my experience with eating.
They were hand in hand.

Overall, I really felt crap.
It's not until something is gone, do you value what it
means to you.
I was on a mission to feel healthy again but had lost
motivation and frankly, I couldn't see the light at the end
of the tunnel.
The one thing on my side was that I *knew* there was a
way out.

There had to be.

I have this stupid comparison I do sometimes, but it actually helps me have confidence in what I want to do. I think to myself "if someone who is living on the streets on drugs, or an alcoholic, can turn their life around, you can".
I know it sounds stupid, but I guess if you think of a person who has all odds against them, and then think of yourself, in a good, clean country, with means, opportunity and a desire to be better, surely I can do it too?
But I digress…

I recall a yoga class whilst in triangle pose feeling a loss of breath and physically not being able to reach my arm down enough. I could feel the flexibility was there, it was the extra roll of 'meat' getting in the way.

Things like this caused a major mess with emotions, because yoga, one of my favourite forms of exercise was now embarrassing. We laid down for corpse pose at the end of the class and I felt the flow pour out of my tear glands. There was no sobbing, just internal sadness looking for a way out.

I remember the internal dialog vividly as the tears poured down my face as I lay in silence.
"I am so sorry, I am sorry, I am so so sorry" - as if another person had been hurting me these years.
Someone separate from me.
Someone who had just realised that the *one* person they should have been treating right was themselves.
I was genuinely so sorry for having hurt *me*.

WHAT I DISCOVERED ABOUT EXERCISE

When you try all the diets, you try all the exercises too.
I loved moving and being fit.

Sometimes, along the way, exercise stops being for fun
and health. It turns into something you do to burn
calories. You say things like, "I will burn that off in the
morning" when your fitness should be unrelated to your
food.
Yes, I wanted to be fit and healthy, but I had turned
exercise into a punishment.
Measuring and creating plans to burn, burn, burn was
my modus operandi.

I love/d exercise, but I had turned something I loved into
an integral part of my eating disorder.
In my journey to heal my eating disorder, I realised I
had to also heal my relationship with exercise.
I always knew that it made me feel good, but it wasn't
until I released the association between calorie burn and
punishment did I remember how much I loved it.

In my reading, research and awakening, I suddenly had
become hypersensitive to the way people spoke about
exercise. The way they had to constantly point out how
much they had done, or how much they *would do* to
burn off calories while they were eating a slice of cake.
The two are mutually exclusive.
You need not burn anything off.
You need to eat well and move well.
Measuring and obsessing turns good health into work
and sometimes, eating disorders.

The other thing I noticed was that people were doing things they didn't like. Outwardly expressing how much they hated a certain exercise.
I felt like screaming "If you don't like it, don't do it"!
There are multiple ways to work a muscle group. If you are trying to get strong legs or increase fitness, find the things you like I say!

When I told a friend I was exercising for fun, she said, "that's cool, not everyone likes to sweat".
That confused me a little, who said I wasn't sweating or having a good workout?
Who said that my *garage workouts* were not good enough for most people?

A stigma comes with working out lately that if you are not training for something, competing in something, or burning something, it's not enough.

"Oh, but you want to know what I'm training for?"
Life.

CHANGING MY BELIEFS ABOUT EXERCISE

Just like with food, I had to make moving fun again.
Without measuring calorie expenditure.

This needed almost the same dedication as I had put towards healing the food side of things.
Although I must admit, this was a lot easier.

My beliefs about exercise had to change.

I was not training for a marathon, I had done that sort of thing before.

I was training for life. Long term.

There was no short-term goal.
I was looking for a long-term sustainable way of life.
Training for a marathon ends, training for life is forever.

I was looking for all the things I loved to do with my body and incorporate them into my life.

Move for fun and feeling good, that was the aim.

This is hard to do outwardly.
Internally I am really OK with this.
I know I am fit and healthy.
I know I am moving my body.
I know I love exercise.

Outwardly, however, I am not talking about a 4-week F45 challenge, or a 6-week boot camp, tough mudder or a marathon I am training for.
You certainly can't see my 6 pack.
But I don't think this means I am not healthy does it? ;)

Because I am not doing these things and talking about my exercise, people *assume* I don't do it.

I have been at a table where someone systematically went around the table asking everyone what they did for fitness and they by-passed me. I can only assume it was because I didn't look fit and slender.

Had they asked me I would have said, I walk every morning, I hike when I can, I drag my hubby on a bike ride when possible, I dance, punch my punching bag or lift weights every afternoon and finish with some yoga. And in summer, I work out in my pool. Yeah, like Aqua Aerobics. No judgment, please.
I'm active.
I'm just not *skinny*.

My beliefs about exercise have changed significantly. From needing fancy equipment, hours of my day, following all the new fads and expensive gym memberships; I now believe that exercise should be fun, tailored to suit what <u>you like</u> and something you can easily do anywhere, with no fancy equipment.
I am training for life. Not an event.
My mind keeps wandering back to the stone age for some reason. I am constantly wondering how on earth people kept fit before Boot Camps and F45 Classes? How did anyone get by? ;)

MY LIFE LESSONS from MOVING AND SHAKING:

- Fitness is not a means to a skinny end
- I love moving my body
- Strong and Flexible is where it is at
- You need not spend much or any money to be fit
- I will never train for an event again. I am fit for life because I love it.
- Fancy equipment and special classes are unnecessary.
- Keep it simple. Nothing is wrong with a good walk.

Chapter 6 – The Tough Stuff

BEING DRIVEN

If you are reading this book, you yourself must be somewhat driven.
There may be something holding you back from believing in yourself, but you must know that if you have reached this point, there is a part of you that wants better; has hope for something better.

Since forever I have always had drive.
It is what kept me on the diet roller coaster.
I was driven to be skinny. My drive didn't get me where I wanted to be. I was barking up the wrong tree.

I am not really the sort of person that takes no for an answer, and I *rarely* don't get what I want.
I don't mean to say that in a cocky way.
I go for what I want and put it out there. I'm not afraid to ask the question.
By default, this means I more frequently get what I want.

It is rare for me to sit there wondering.
That has to be attributed to my mummy's voice ringing in my head from when I was a kid. "Always ask questions, only ignorant people don't ask questions".
The other thing she would always say was "It's better to ask and get a no than to miss out on a yes for lack of trying".

My mum was basically telling me to 'ask for the sale'.

Even when I was 19, I had the attitude that if I wanted something, I could search the yellow pages and find it… these days, it's Google.

So what does being driven mean? Why does it matter?
Well, I have always known deep down inside that things
can get better.
I was not meant to live an average life. A peaceful life,
yes. But not average.
I would never sit back and let problems defeat me. I
would break the walls down and have a better life.

I absolutely could have continued dieting forever. It's
not like this is unheard of. I have heard 70-year-old
women talking about their diets. It is totally feasible;
almost socially acceptable. But why would I want that?

Why would anybody want that?

When we have a life in front of us, filled with
possibilities, adventures to be had, people to help, love
to give; why would I spend my time worrying about the
way I look alone?

Yes, I should spend time on the way I feel and being
healthy, but if I don't have a 6 pack, is that really the
end of the world? Is that really where I hold my value in
life?
No. It's not. Because if it was, I would have done that by
now.

My drive lies in wanting to experience all the great
things this life has to offer, and I don't have *hating
myself* on that list.

Hating and torturing myself is not what I want in life.

Being driven means you know there is better for you and you go for it.
Even when you can't see a way out, you just don't give up.
Even now, I know there is still work to be done. It is constant.
I will continue practicing <u>conscious</u> self-love and self-care forever.
So, 30 plus years of hurting myself proves that self-care does not come naturally.
I clearly have a pre-disposition to play the 'you are not good enough' game.
I know I must try to love myself forever.

But honestly, that is not a chore.
Self-love and self-care are always good. 'Me' time is not a punishment.
Reflection and growing as a human are not painful.
It's necessary. And now, often my favourite thing.

IF I QUIT DIETS, AM I GOING TO BE FAT?

I am not a dietitian, nor am I a clairvoyant, so I don't think I or most other people could answer that accurately for you.

I can understand your fear though. You could even read my story, thinking, this isn't very inspirational, she packed on the kilos and is telling me if I follow what she did, I will be fatter!
Hold up… we haven't gotten to my 'happily ever after' yet.

If you do what I did in the order I did it, then the

likelihood of you putting on weight is high.
But that is kinda the point of this book.
I suffered so much that I wanted to share my mistakes to
inspire others to do things differently.
Do the right things I did, but a year earlier. Or do them
now!

If I did all the things I have done to heal as soon as I quit
diets, rather than 1 year later, I would have <u>likely</u> not put
on the weight that I did.
I was unprepared.

Everyone is different, not me, nor any professional can
predict what will happen to you.

You may have only dieted for a few years and not tried
everything I have tried, you may be in a worse position
and need immediate professional help.
Everyone is different.

Just get prepared.

IT'S HARD

I am not about to ~~stevia~~ sugar coat it.
The journey is hard. The struggle *is* real.
If creating a sustainable life of health is what you are
looking for then it is <u>more</u> than worth it.

And hey, you may be tougher than me. I could be a
flouncy weaky weakington for all you know.
You might be made of a little more concrete than me.

There will be times where you question your decision and your methods.
Sometimes, you hear about a diet and think, 'just one more' (to get a few kilos off).
There may be times when you think you need to re-install myfitnesspal and start counting calories again because if you could only track them, you could make sure you were not eating too much.
You will think, 'If only I could just weigh myself to see if I had lost weight!'

I have been there.
And it wasn't just once.
I took a long time to break the habits of a dieter.
They still pop into my head occasionally. I have just learned how to respond with common sense and remember my values when using my inner dialog back to the former dieter in me.

Why does the number on the scale matter?
What matters is this:

Do I feel good?
Yes! (Keep going). No (Change things up. Something isn't working).

I learned to use my instincts. Like they did in the olden days. A thing like that!
I had to let go of all the *numbers* I was using to measure my success and replace them all with my feelings and my 'gut'.

Here is what I swapped out:
-Scales: The number didn't matter as long as I was

feeling healthier.

-Pedometer/Fitness Tracker: as long as I was moving every day, it didn't matter what the little device had to say I was winning by moving.

-Clothing size: I cut the tags off and only wore clothes that fit well or were loose. If clothing was tight I would feel down on myself and that was not conducive to healing and feeling good about myself.

- Calorie Counting: This was unnecessary. I was eating good food at meal times. If I felt full I had eaten too much and would know to eat less next time.

But remember, this would not have been possible without a massive change in mindset.

IS IT HARD ON YOUR RELATIONSHIPS?

I found my relationships suffered when I was at the peak of my eating disorder.

I was not myself, largely because I was taking prescription diet pills which were messing with my head.

I didn't feel like myself. I didn't feel proud of myself and didn't love myself.

You know what they say if you don't love yourself, how can anyone else?

Luckily, my now hubby didn't get the memo on that one.

He continued to love me fiercely and help me any way he could.

I was not the nicest person when I was going through the peak of my disorder or recovery. I was down on myself and would take it out on the one I loved most.

My husband has zero concept of what it's like to have an eating disorder. He cannot relate in the slightest. I would never have told him this at the time, but his lack of 'relatability' was just what I needed.
His level-headedness and matter of fact approach to health are so simple.
Simple is what I needed.
His advice and kind words helped me through.

My issues also affected other relationships. I didn't want to be a bridesmaid because I was at the start of my journey and didn't want to put off my recovery for an event that would be a major trigger. This made me the most petrified.

I kept things from friends and basically was not my authentic self.

I kept a part of myself secret from so many people…

Since reaching the place where I sit happily now, I am pleased to say that friendships are stronger than ever.
It is amazing how much better your friendships are when you are yourself.

MY LIFE LESSONS from WHEN THE TOUGH STUFF:

- Nothing will work unless you do
- Drive is everything
- If you will make a massive life change, be prepared.
    Call for help!
- Anything that makes me track my progress with a
    number to validate my worth
is kiboshed.
- Telling people was the best thing I did

Chapter 7 – Doubling Down

THE LONG GAME

I've never been a fan of The Long Game.
I have always been a here and now, get it done, I want it yesterday kinda gal.
In hindsight, I wasn't a fan of The Long Game because I had never tried it.
I was ignorant of its efficacy in some situations.

My Hubby is the one who taught me The Long Game.
He would see me in pain and keep telling me it would take years to achieve certain goals and that it was OK for it to take that long.
But I didn't want to believe him.
In my heart, I wanted to be better instantly. I didn't understand how *years* would help.
I thought I just needed to be tough and have willpower and have an instant change in mindset.
But he was right. So that's why I dedicate this section especially to him.
To say thanks…and babe, you were right.
There are so many things that had to change inside my mind to go from being 'here and now Kelly' to playing 'The Long Game Kelly'.
I didn't want things to take *long*. I wanted to be fixed now!
But doing the same things repeatedly and expecting different results is the definition of insanity, right?
Nothing is wrong with doing things quickly. I still am that person, but having now experienced such a wonderful eye-opening journey, I see there is a time and a place for both ways.
Is there something you have always wanted to do that you keep trying and keep failing at?

Here is some *food for thought* that may help you break those old patterns and set your Long Game up for success:
Think of that 'something' you want and haven't achieved, be it a material possession, your mindset, your body, or a relationship….
If you have spent years 'failing' at achieving this *thing*, wouldn't it be OK to dedicate 1-3 years <u>slowly</u> working on it to make long-lasting change? Do you want to be 70 and think, if I had only done *this* or only tried *that*??

If you keep doing what you have done nothing will change. You must keep trying different approaches till something works.
We live in a world where we want things instantly, but just like coffee, the instant stuff never tastes as good.
The bean carefully grown, in loving conditions, handpicked, roasted, properly stored, then brewed to perfection is the stuff we like best.
So why would it be any different for our lives? (maybe because we are not a coffee bean, but you know what I mean!)

And in my case, it was better to read, learn, talk, and try lots of different things to achieve what I wanted, rather than to think I could be different overnight and instantly just have all new habits and beliefs.
For me, I had to really learn about everything I needed to heal and change my mindset.
Slow and Steady wins the race.

YOUR MINDSET HAS TO CHANGE

Because this isn't a quick process you must be OK with playing the *long game*.
You must dig deep inside and understand that Rome wasn't built in a day. All the great things in life take time.
Quick fixes and 4-week programs do not build Rome. They build a pop-up cafe in your local city center that can be torn down in a day.
Do you want to be torn down in a day, or do you want to create long-lasting beauty that will be admired for a lifetime?

A lot had to change for me to embrace a new way of life.
It wasn't as simple as eating better, loving yourself more and taking better care of yourself.

I had to truly believe that making this change was going to be the best thing.

I had to somehow stop believing that skinny was better. I know there are a few different 'camps' when it comes to how a woman should feel about her body these days.

There is a very obvious online influencer community of people sending the message, of *'nothing tastes as good as skinny feels'. Skinny is best, etc. (this is the camp I had lived in for most of my life).*

Then there is the other end of the spectrum.
Love who you are, big is beautiful. Who cares what you look like, it's what's inside that counts.
I have tried to sit in this camp, teetered on the edge of

hanging out here, but never stuck around for long.

Finally, there is the camp which I believe sits
somewhere in the middle.
Yes. I am a fence sitter.
I love all people of every size, having been lots of sizes,
I can attest to my being equally as lovable at each
juncture, however…
I think *you* need to do *you*.

Someone should not be shamed for being
overweight(because you have no idea what they have
been through or *are* going through).
But I also don't think someone should be shamed for
wanting to look after themselves either.

I took a while to figure out my beliefs on this.

My immediate reaction when I realised I needed to quit
dieting and love myself more was to do a complete
back-flip.
I was very righteous and wanting to embrace my body
and love myself. And eat anything I wanted.
I started thinking to myself, 'Who cares what other
people think about me, as long as I am happy, that's all
that should matter.
But this didn't sit right with me.
I didn't want to let myself go and not care about myself.
I love good healthy food and would choose roast veggies
over a pizza any day of the week. I would have a nice
salad over a big mac any given Sunday.
And I love exercise and feeling fit.
I have done exercise all my life and feel a substantial
difference when I don't do it. Mentally and Physically.

So, going to the other extreme didn't feel right.
Even if it was the obvious first choice to make a stand;
to make up for the years of self-hatred.

I had to do a lot of reading, listening, and self-reflection
to finally understand where my values were.
I didn't want to let myself go. I still cared about staying
a size that made me feel comfortable.
And I don't mean a dress size or a number on the scale.
I mean waking up in the morning and feeling fit, feeling
healthy, getting dressed and liking the reflection.

I had to learn to love what I saw.
This was me. Warts and all.

I had to understand that everyone has *something* they
think is wrong with them.
This realisation opened my eyes to the fact that if we all
think we have something wrong with us, aren't we all
perfectly imperfect?

You have big ears, but a thin waist. She has a beautiful
face and a solid build. He has great muscles and he is
short.
And that's just the physical. Let's blend this theory with
personality…
He has a great face but is mean. She is so funny and
lovable but has thinning hair.

Nobody is perfect. We are all perfectly imperfect.

When you truly understand this, all of a sudden, your so-
called imperfections are just something you have, to
balance out the rest of your perfectness!

WABI-SABI

Japanese culture has something called Wabi-Sabi.
Basically, it means that we should look at the world as
perfect imperfection.
Nothing lasts, nothing is perfect.

Wabi refers to the simplicity of something, manmade or
natural. As well as any 'defects' that add to the
uniqueness and beauty of something.

Sabi is the beauty that comes with age.

When I look at myself I think Wabi-Sabi, when I look at
you I think Wabi-Sabi.
We are all perfectly imperfect in our own ways and my
imperfection could very well be your strength and vice
versa.

Learning things such as the above, really opened my
eyes to the fact that there was no reason to hate on
myself for anything.
If I am always doing my best, then I am always proud.

Let's take this book for example.
I have no idea if it will be an awesome book in the eyes
of millions of people, or even hundreds of people.
I will do my best.
I know I enjoy writing it.
Will it be perfect?
It will be perfectly imperfect for me.

I had to apply Wabi Sabi to every thought process so I
could understand that I am perfectly imperfect in every

way.

My mindset had to change so much so, that I had to adore me. More than anything else.
When I did this my whole life changed.

I now prioritise *me* over anything else, any day of the week.

Take my day job, I love it. But I love me more.
If I need to go for a massage, exercise or do anything else that feeds my soul I will do it right after work, rather than working late and not caring for myself.

Once, I would work most nights and miss out on these things.
Now I strive for balance.
I go hard during the day. I will barely take a personal call if I am working.
When 5 or 6 pm comes along I (mostly) know it's <u>time for me</u>.
I need this. I need to feed my soul.
Of course, there are times where I will work all night If I am working on something important, but if it can wait I know that my self-care is my number 1 priority.

I had to change the way my mind worked; which took me to a place of always trying to be something better and hating myself for not being it; to finding all the amazing things within me and nurturing those things with passion.
That goes for most things in life. The more you focus on something, the more it grows.
If I am spending most of my time looking at the best in

me, the best in me grows.
The same theory applies to other people in your life.
You can spend your whole time hating someone or
pointing out their flaws, but when you focus on what is
great about them, their greatness shines!

Only once I finally loved and accepted myself, was I
able to get on with the rest of it; and by the *rest of it*, I
mean the job of restoring my relationship with food and
fitness.
The trial and error of finding what foods I actually liked,
disliked, didn't want to have much of, took a while to
figure out.

Realising that my 'food' project, also included a mind-
body-soul focus, was what took a high-level project into
what I believe was a deeper more authentic healing.

HOW I DEALT WITH EVENTS

Making the choice to change your life can be very
exciting and almost feels like it will be easy once you
have made your mind up.

Things pop-up that will catch you by surprise. Things
you may not have thought of.
I had to think on my feet and not lose sight of my goal.

The major challenge was events.
'Events' was a really tough one because of three things,
my clothing, seeing people I hadn't seen in a while and
actually participating in activities.

The key to my success at events was to go all in!

First, I had to dress for the occasion. I made sure I had good fitting clothing I was comfortable in.
I incorporated a few little psychological tricks to make me feel good too; as I mentioned previously, I cut the tag off my clothing so I couldn't see the size.
I didn't want to look at a size and feel down about any weight I had gained. I removed any obstacles to my healing to ensure I would feel good, as often as possible.
I knew that if my mind was good, the rest would follow.
I would make sure my clothing made me feel good, even if it meant I spent a little more than usual on an item.
If I felt good, that was all that mattered.
I had a laser focus on making myself better and would do anything to achieve this.

Seeing people I hadn't seen in a while was a tough one.
Especially once I had put on the 25kg.
I thought their eyes would pop out of their heads when they saw me.
They didn't.
They didn't say a word, not in front of me anyway.
Then I thought to myself; 'who cares, if they say anything, they don't know me, they don't know my journey and how all-consuming this has been'.
If someone doesn't know your full story (which many people would not), they really can't judge you on the real you.
Only you can do that.
If I was proud of myself, then that was all that mattered.

Participating in activities was something I was still a little selective on.

I now will not shy away from activities like I used to, and I try to say things to myself like, 'would you do that if you were 10 kilos lighter? If so, then do it. Why should I miss out!
I didn't miss out on anything, but I wasn't about to go swimming with my work colleagues. There are some things most people would draw the line on. :)

PREPARING FOR QUITTING DIETS

Before I tell you about what I would have done differently when I quit diets, I must say this…
I know *people* say you should 'have no regrets'; and really, I don't.
But let's say I had a daughter in the same situation, and I wanted to prevent her some pain, or if I had a best friend who could learn from my mistakes; would I tell them to do things differently?
YES.
I don't look at that as regret. I see it as wisdom to not make the same mistake twice.

If I had my time over, once I had decided to quit diets I would have done it with the help and guidance of a professional.
Like I did 18 months in.
I would do everything just the same, only earlier.

About 18 months into quitting diets, I hadn't figured out how to eat like a normal person. I had given myself binge eating disorder.
It started by deciding to 'treat myself' for everything I had been missing out on… and that turned into what I feel was an addiction.

I was particularly addicted to anything sugary or pastry-like.
I am not normally drawn to bread or pastry type products, I don't mind them occasionally, but this became an unhealthy, unbalanced fixation.
It felt like an addiction. It was uncontrollable. It wasn't pretty.
I literally felt like a junkie, but for croissants.
I would make myself sick and have stomach aches so fierce that I was almost in tears.
Even after one bite, I couldn't breathe.
My whole body felt puffy and broken.
Puff Pastry stayed true to its name.

I thought I wasn't going on a diet when I quit diets, but I was still mentally on one.
Mentally, I wasn't letting myself have anything sweet, and I was trying to restrict certain things. But physically, I was rewarding myself for a lifetime of deprivation.
It was much more subtle and there was no diet plan I had written on a piece of paper, but I was still trying to deprive myself of things, which would cause these binges.

If I had my time over I would speak to a professional (such as a psychologist or specialist in eating disorders) about what I was hoping to do and have guidance and help along the way.
I would have worked on my self-love on day one; as a priority.

The day I returned from my honeymoon, and the diets were over, I would have gone to a professional and told

them I was sick of going on diets and I was not looking to lose weight *fast* anymore.
I would tell them I have been dieting all my life and have just been on a few nasty ones over the last six months and I needed help weaning off them and restoring my body to health.
I would tell them I wanted to do this with moderation and finding techniques to assist me with this transition.
I would tell them about the fact that I had not felt good about the way I was treating myself and I needed help.
I would have been prepared to take specialist referrals to help me through this in a healthy way.

The years after quitting diets were the most rewarding, but also what I feel was 'rock bottom'.
I had quit but didn't know how to be 'normal'.

MY LIFE LESSONS from DOUBLING DOWN:

- I love the long game. Effort and patience equal a massive reward here.
- Listen to your husband.
- Willpower has nothing to do with a mental issue surrounding food.
- It was all in my head. Literally. Working on my mind was key to my recovery.
- Googling the crap out of the free resources available to us was my best friend.
- We are all perfectly imperfect
- Love and acceptance of one's self is all a person should ever wish for
- Me-time is real. I need it. It is as essential as air.
- Wearing clothes that make me feel good can get me through any event.

Chapter 8 – All the Stuff I Did Right

I DID A LOT RIGHT!

I have told you all the things I did wrong, but I did a lot right too!

When I finally hit rock bottom, I was away for work, in a job I hated. I had no idea what I had done to my body or my career. In turn, I was being a horrible, needy wife. Winging and 'down' all the time.
I was desperately unhappy.

I remember calling my husband.
I was in Southern New South Wales, sitting outside of a customer's office in my car, bawling my eyes out.
I felt like I was selling my soul, doing something I didn't love.
I had let myself go and was the unhealthiest I had been in forever.
I had never been so unfit, heavy or down on myself.

A once positive Kelly was a Debbie Downer.
I was desperate, not wanting to ever go on a diet again, but also couldn't handle feeling this way.

I needed to speak to someone(something I should have done immediately, but hey, you live and learn!).
I googled Eating disorders and Psychologists.

The thing to note when looking for a professional to help you with something is this:
You are not always going to connect with everyone.
Just picking a psychologist and seeing them for 10 weeks is not always the way to go.
You are putting your life and money in their hands,

kinda. (You obviously still have all the control, but you don't want to be wasting your money on someone you don't connect with.)

Doing all the research I did and actually finding someone that gave me genuine hope from the first conversation was key. I felt cared for, understood and like this was absolutely the right choice.

My inner guidance system was telling me she was 'the one'.

Funnily enough, she also shared my name (spelt differently).

I found someone in Brisbane, who was not only a specialist in this arena but had a story which read as a replica of mine.

Here was a professional who not only specialised in binge eating and food addiction, but she had walked the path.

She knew exactly what it felt like.

I called her. Immediately.

When she called me back, she gave me a good chunk of her time on the phone and that conversation cemented the idea this woman was for me.

She was warm, real and genuinely sounded like she wanted to help me.

I had tried talking to psychologists before. But nothing as specialised as this.

I hadn't spoken with anyone that I felt would genuinely get in deep and help me get to the *root of the problem*.

I DIDN'T GIVE UP

Once I found Kellee, I didn't instantly get better.
It took time. She helped me uncover a lot about myself.

Confidence in myself and change of mindset was the
main thing we worked on.
You hear it all the time, but seriously, nothing is more
powerful than healing your mind.

It was hard, sometimes I didn't feel like I was ever
going to 'get better' but I just kept trying.
I just knew I could do it. I thought if an alcoholic or
drug addict can turn their life around, surely I can?
With all the resources and possibilities I had at my
disposal, surely??

I didn't understand <u>why</u> I was doing <u>what</u> I was doing.
We looked at everything from childhood to the more
recent goings on in my life.

We found the 'why' and the triggers and then worked on
how to overcomes these.
Mainly with kindness to myself.
Kellee was very good at giving me that virtual 'smack
on the hand' when I wasn't being kind to myself.

Even after I felt there was an obvious 'stop point' to my
visits with Kellee, I kept working on things myself at
home to ensure I was giving myself the care and love I
needed.
I kept reading books and trying to find my version of
healthy.

They are not wrong when they say it's the journey, not the destination.
I haven't woken up one day and thought, 'Oh, I am healed now'.

It's actually much better than that. It is the journey itself, the daily up's and down's and figuring things out for yourself which gives you the satisfaction.
It is the soul-searching and epiphanies… the light bulb moments that give you the most satisfaction.

The most beautiful part is the fierce love affair you create with yourself. That moment when you realise <u>you</u> have been the lioness of your life; it's what makes you most proud.

TRIAL AND ERROR.

There was no 'answer' per se.

There was a hell of a lot of trial and error. I took a long time to figure out what I feel is now a great self-lovin-lifestyle.

Sometimes I tried to do things too systematically. To rigidly.
Other times I was too relaxed.

I tried to plan out my day, attempt to follow the plan and then beat myself up for not doing this perfectly.
I often tried to weave in the rigidity I had with diets, feeling that's what was needed. But this never worked.

Luckily, my mummy taught me to always ask why???
If something wasn't working, I would always ask why??
Then try something else.
I would brainstorm what was wrong with my plan and
try and make a change.

One thing highlighted by the discovery work I had been
doing was that I would turn to food when I was anxious
or unhappy.

I wasn't doing any of the things I loved or **fed my soul**.
So instead, I had fed my mouth.

I guess all people need various amounts of soul-feeding,
and this work uncovered I need lots.

If someone asked me to describe what I love and feeds
my soul, the answer would be something like this:

'I love life and want to try <u>everything</u> it has to offer.
I need to create and love to write, paint and draw.
I want to help the world. I am a conscious human, and
although not perfect, I try to do things to help our earth.
I want to help others.
I love to move my body, be in nature, hike, swim, beach,
and bike.
I want to Daaaaaaance. (I am sure I was a dancer in my
past life. I had always wanted to be a dancer but didn't
go through with it at the final hour because I didn't think
my body was good enough.)
Finally, I want to give and love!'

Do you know how much of that soul food I was doing in

the lead to my lowest point?
None.
Actually, that's a lie. We completed the Oxfam
trailwalker hike in that time.
Other than that, there was nothing else.

I figured out all the things I needed to make me happy
and feed my soul, and once this happened, I didn't need
to feed myself!
(Well, of course, I fed myself, but for normal
nourishment, not to fill some sort of void.)

I have heard people say that if you fill yourself with the
things you love, there will be no room for the things that
have not been serving you.
It played out exactly like that.

WHAT A CLICHÉ!

This is so cliché, but it's probably the most important
part.
Every time I 'fell down' I got back up again.

As I said before, there was no magic date in the calendar
I can call my anniversary of being healed.

It was literally like this diagram below:

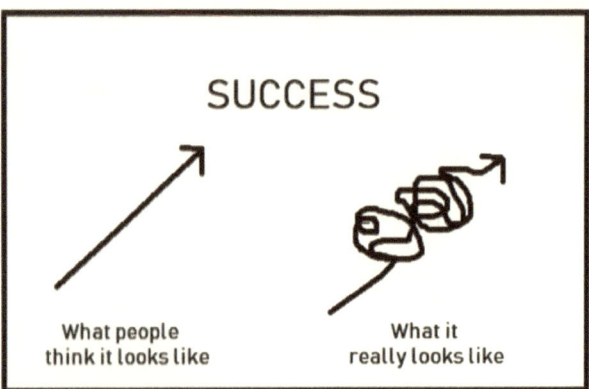

And it still is that way!

One time I fell into a little hole for about two weeks, a hole I thought I could get out of myself. After two weeks I reached out to my hubby and told him I needed some help. We had a good chat and he reminded me of what I already knew about the key to my healing (but couldn't see) and got my mind back to a good place. The key was to not let the 'down' moments take over. I could not stay in the 'hole'.
In the above example, the day I felt like I had lost sight of my journey I tried to fix it myself, seven days in I still tried to fix it myself. On day 14 when I was clearly not figuring it out on my own, I reached out to my hubby, had that great chat and he helped me understand what I was doing wrong. I had been trying to deprive myself for an event again (subconsciously) and this had caused me to feel negative and want to overeat.
As soon I restored everything back to a place of self-love and care (not deprivation), I felt healthy and happy again.

Now I know that if I fall, I can try and fix it myself, but if I can't figure it out on my own, I need to reach out for help.
Two weeks is my limit.
I can't let things drag on for months in the hope I can figure it out on my own. Reaching out for help and nipping anything in the bud is like having a coach to get you back on track.

A WINNING ATTITUDE

I have mentioned this a few times, but I will touch on it again as it was one of the most important aspects of my recovery and the thing I am most proud of.

In this process, I realised this was my life which I was sculpting. I would not keel over and let it pass me by.
I didn't want to wake up one day realising I had lived a life hating myself the whole time.

Imagine waking up on your 90th birthday next to a man who had emotionally abused you your whole life and never having had the courage to leave and change anything.

That is what I feared, but worse.
It wasn't another person hurting me. It was me!
I have 100% control over myself. And luckily, I have the most loving and supportive husband.
I didn't want to wake up at 90 and think, "Wow, you have been unkind and hated yourself for all of your life. You have lived a life where you were never quite good

enough. You have looked in the mirror every day and hated what you have seen."

That was not something I wanted to experience.
I am with me 100% of the time and I have 100% control over me.
Why the hell would I want to spend a second not being 100% kind and true to myself?

I understand that in my life I may be in situations where I feel hurt by another human being.
But I would not be that person hurting myself!

If I can be cocky and not at all humble for a moment, I would like to profess my undying love for myself and say that my desire to love and care for myself like a fierce lioness is what I am most proud of, and what I love most about myself.

I feel that was my secret, winning ingredient.

DEALING WITH COMPLIMENTS

There was one thing that made me uncomfortable and very anxious.
It's something that was said that I feel need not be said or praised as if I have just won an Archibald Prize.
A customer said, "You look so tiny".
Me, thinking she meant short, replied, "What do you mean?"
She said, "You look so skinny".
First, I weighed 78kg. I was not *so skinny*, so my mind went to all these places:

Why do you have to comment on my weight?
How massive did I look before? (I had dropped one
dress size)
I am not *skinny*.
Why does society need to comment on what I look like,
there is so much more to be said.

From once being a person that needed and wanted to be
thin, I now struggled to take a compliment for
something I didn't think should be complimented.
Now I love myself for who I am, the outside is so
irrelevant. I want to be healthy, whatever that looks like.

After this 'compliment' happened, I also felt very
anxious all day.
I didn't even put 2 and 2 together till I realised the
afternoon snack I ate was emotionally driven, rather than
from hunger.
So, once I figured the two events were related, in true
Kelly style, I had to analyse the crap out of it.
I didn't want a compliment to throw me off my path to
recovery.
Even my lovely man tried to assist in launching the
epiphany but to no avail.
Not until a few days after did I find a way to be at peace
with what she had said
At a visit, my psychologist was trying to unpack what
had happened and she asked me, "What do you feel
proud of"?
My answer was this:
*"I have been working hard to embed a good routine into
my life, daily walking, meditation, good herbs, self-love,
keeping hydrated, moving my body, art and getting good
sleep.*

Doing things that make me smile and caring for myself;
Giving myself so much love.
I have not been trying to lose weight. I have not been
excessively exercising, counting steps or calories. I can
feel I have lost weight very slowly as a by-product but
mainly, I have been trying to be my true self and do
things that make me happy and healthy and it has
worked."

Who would have thought that living an authentic life
would have made you happy and healthy?
(massive sarcasm intended)

She told me that next time someone commented or paid
a compliment, to imagine they were praising me for my
organisation and my greatness in living such an
authentic life.

You should have seen my body language and a massive
smile emerge at that point!!
I was elated. Smiling ear to ear.
"I can totally accept praise for that!" I said

THAT is what I am proud of.
That is what I have been striving for.
Not Kilos. Kilos on or off didn't make me happy.
It was living a life I was proud of that made me happy.
AND I AM PROUD!!! (Sorry for shouting.)
She gave me a few tools to keep up my sleeve.
Next time someone asks me if I have lost weight, I will
imagine they are praising the things I am proud of, and
the sustainable lifestyle I have created.
Rather than my appearance. (This will make me smile
because I am happy to take praise for that.)

And, I will say this:

Thanks for noticing! ...then swiftly change the topic to something more interesting.

And If they pay me a compliment, I will again imagine what I am proud of and say:

"I appreciate that"

People obviously mean no harm when they pay a compliment... but for *weirdos* like me who feel strongly against such compliments, this technique helps me find the *good* in the situation.

I HAD A GOAL

I was excited to turn 40. I did not understand why. But I was. I had good vibes about 40.

They say it's when life begins, but I don't know about that.

I feel like I have squashed more adventure, laughter, good times, fun, mistakes, wins, sadness, and happiness into my life than I could have ever dreamed!

I will take a stab in the dark, but I think more so than life beginning, in the next 40 years I will get to put all my experience and wisdom into action and give so much to this life and world.

Do it all again so to speak, just a little smarter.

And there will be more wins, mistakes and sadness, happiness and of course adventure, fun, and laughter.

But it will be felt and lived through the wisdom and appreciation of someone who has done a lot of it before.

I feel I have achieved everything I ever wanted and more and achieving doesn't mean owning things, it means feeling things, knowing things and being where I want to be in life mentally.

I had one little goal for 40.
OK, a MASSIVE goal which was that I didn't want to have major issues with an eating disorder and I wanted to have a semblance of a good relationship with food.

One thing I learned was that reaching my goal was not what I thought. I thought my whole mind would be different and I would be like the people who have never had an eating disorder.
It's not like that. If you are like me, you will never have that.
You will have something BETTER.
You will have compassion and understanding for anyone with similar issues.
You will have the knowledge it is always there but you will own it.

Excuse my language, but it's the only way I know how to say:
When you get to this point, your eating disorder no longer owns you. You own it.
It is your bitch! You tell it what to do. You tell it how to behave. It is there, but it sits oh so quietly in the corner while its authoritarian boss-lady (you) tells it what to do. And that, my friends, feels so much better than anything I could have ever imagined.

That was my goal and I am proud to say it was achieved with flying colours.

I LOOKED AFTER MYSELF. BIG TIME.

I mentioned this a little earlier, everyone requires different levels of Self-Care.
Some people are born with that cup of concrete in their hand. Others need a little care and others need a lot more.
We shouldn't try and walk around with the cup of concrete just because others do. (as much as I have tried, that tactic has not worked)
We must give ourselves the love we require.
We are all made up of different things, we've all had different life experience and different upbringings.
You know you better than anyone.
You know if you need a weekly coffee with girlfriends, a long bath at the end of the week, a regular yoga practice or all the above.
Or you may need nothing at all. (You're made of concrete.)

I believe everyone has a path. It's the thing in your heart that tells you the sort of person you are, the things you love, the things that make your heart sing, your values, and your dreams.
When you are young, you head off on a journey, doing the things you love and being the person you are.
Occasionally, you veer off your path because you must focus on other things.
These 'other things' are not necessarily bad or good…

You may meet new friends with different interests, a new partner, lose loved ones, find a new job, change career or have children…
Each time you face these changes, getting back onto your original path may seem difficult and one day you realise you are no longer doing the things you once loved and made you very happy.

This, in fact, happened to me. I had stopped doing the things that made me happy. It wasn't anyone's fault. Life changes happened rapidly and suddenly, I was not doing anything that fed my soul.

In my recovery, I did lots of exploring to find what was important and made time for them. They were necessary. They were a must.

To ensure I was incorporating something in my day that meant I was caring for myself, I created a Self-Care Planner which I now use daily. It is not a rigid planner. I merely have suggestions here to guide me throughout my day.

The image on the following page depicts the part of the book I use daily, but I also house in here a section for affirmations and a few other little helpful messages for when I need them.
I fill this in every day and it has helped me with restoring my self-confidence and love for myself.

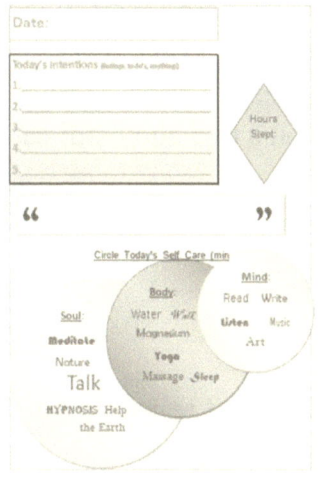
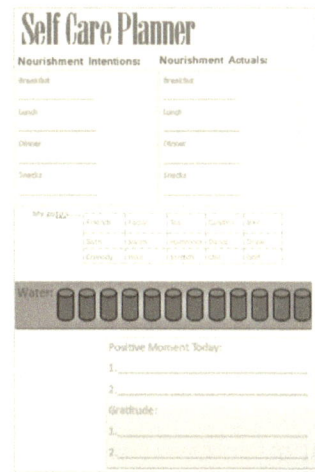

How do I use this?

I keep it open just as shown in the study next to where I keep my devices charging.

Every morning I fill in most of it. It takes a minute to write a few lines down and circle what self-care I will incorporate into my day.

It's designed to set the intentions for my day and remind me of the things I would like to do, to ensure I am keeping my 'cup full'.

At night I fill in the bottom sections about gratitude and water. Again, it takes only a min.

What's the purpose?

It keeps me positive and on track with achieving what I must do in a day to keep me happy and healthy.

Evidently, I need a planner to do this because I am easily distracted and need help with focus sometimes.

Other people may be able to use their brain alone ;)

I LISTENED TO MY BODY, AND IT SPOKE LOUD AND CLEAR

Now, I must be clear, I am not on a diet and I still eat most foods occasionally.
Through trial and error, there were certain foods that I found to not be helpful or didn't make me feel good.
As my recovery was all about feeling good, I needed to 86 a few things that weren't serving me.

As I sunk my teeth into my recovery, I learned a lot about myself.
I had up's and down's in the process; because at times I just felt like I didn't know if I would figure out how to eat normally.
I struggled with ever going on a diet again, but I so desperately wanted to stop the binging. I kept having thoughts about 'one last diet'. I felt I couldn't get control over certain foods and I just couldn't figure out how to make it work.

I was very torn between two ideas I was having.
One was that I wanted to learn to eat ALL things in moderation; then there was the other part of me that strongly believed that certain foods caused an addiction type of response in me.

I read a lot about addiction, food addiction in particular, and I remember in that moment feeling totally at peace.
Like I had uncovered the treasure. The missing piece of the puzzle.
I knew this was the breakthrough I had been looking for.

Apparently, there is no such diagnosis as 'Food Addiction', I have obviously never gone to a doctor who has run tests on me. But I am the 'experimental scientist of my life'.

And I am certain that a few foods cause a chemical reaction inside of me that swayed me to eat them excessively, in one sitting without control or thought. They cause all the same responses and feeling as an alcoholic would have and in turn create just as much pain.

So, with that said, there are a few ingredients that I don't eat for two reasons, they make me feel like crap, and they have caused a little bit of an addiction trigger. No amount of mindfulness or intuitive eating techniques can help me with these ingredients.

I don't restrict my eating in any way. There are just a few ingredients that I 'swap out' to make me feel good after eating.

I still eat whatever I feel like, except a few ingredients I see as my drug.

For the first time in my life, I feel free and happy. My insides feel A-M-A-Z-I-N-G. I have never felt like this EVER before.

I previously stopped myself from eating certain dishes. I no longer do this. I simply swap out a few ingredients for alternatives that make me feel good and continue with the recipe.

And now I no longer have uncontrollable binge sessions.

And this is how I came up with what I like to call 'Moderation with a Twist'.

Ah! The light bulb moment! <3

I have one little exception; I found there to be one
activity I loved doing with my hubby I just didn't want
to give up. And so far, so good.
I have been able to continue with this activity without it
causing any triggers.

My hubby and I LOVE going to degustation dinners.
We go to them a couple of times per year.

For anyone who has never been to one, they are the tiny
little meals artfully crafted and every morsel is like an
explosion of love in your mouth.
The experience normally lasts 3-4 hours and they serve
anything from 8 – 15 courses which may come with
wine pairings.
This is something I look at as a 'foodie experience'.
These chefs are artists and it's amazing watching all the
creative ways they put ingredients together.
For me, a birthday party is not about the food, it's about
the celebration with friends and family. As is Christmas.
I still get to eat everything I want, minus a few
ingredients.

A degustation dinner is all about art through food and a
treasured experience between my husband and me.
And because of all this, I just take it as it comes. I eat
the full experience.
We go to dinner almost weekly, but degustation dinners
are the only times where I don't care about the
ingredients.
I will not tell an artist to paint differently just for me. :)

They use such tiny amounts of the ingredients on my 'addiction trigger list' that eating them once in a blue moon doesn't make me feel bad.

I feel like I must finish this section with a massive disclaimer.
This is my truth. Not my advice.
There are many people who could learn to manage all ingredients well. I have worked on my 'food project' for so long, with so many professionals and so much trial and error I know this is my truth right now.
Who knows what the future holds, maybe one day when I master intuitive eating I may change things up; But right now, I feel more at peace and happy with my decision to eat the way I do than ever in my life.

I am a massive advocate of intuitive eating and eating in moderation. And my intuition is strongly speaking telling me to never diet again, and eat all things, sans a few ingredients.
This works and I never feel restricted.
I feel empowered.

I CHANGED MY OUTFIT

Talking about clothing feels like a superficial thing to worry about regarding health when there are other important things in the world to be spoken about.
The reason I feel I must spend a little time on this is that when your weight fluctuates month to month, clothing does too.
There are ways I found to manage this piece of the puzzle, so I could get on with healing my health.

Here are some ways that clothing added to the pain of my eating disorder:

Having your 'favourite pair of jeans' is not something you just do when you can't fit into them three months later.
Buying clothes is not something you enjoy when you look at an item and you are constantly thinking 'will this fit me in a months' time? Will I gain weight? Lose weight? Is this a waste of money?
Will that nice dress I want to buy have to go to the local thrift store in six months?
Do I even feel 'me' wearing it? Or am I buying it because it is the only one that fits me in the store?
Clothing was often chosen in one way for me: It fit. My personal style was out the window. I didn't even feel like me. I felt I was in someone else's costume, forced to walk in 'another woman's shoes' so to speak.

Another embarrassing moment with clothing was when I was going out with my husband, and with a wardrobe full of clothing I said, "I have nothing to wear".
I wasn't being a 'stereotypical girl' complaining about wanting more clothing. I literally found myself with a wardrobe full and nothing fit.
I needed to buy a whole new wardrobe.
This was so embarrassing. Especially in front of the person you want to feel most sexy around.
I felt my outside did not reflect my inside.

Once, I read something great that helped me;

Apparently, if you feel unhealthy, it is hard to stop feeling this way if you are wearing ill-fitting clothing.
I found this great advice.
Granted, spending the money on new clothing was not something I wanted to do, but I started feeling like a normal person when my clothing fit me, rather than inching my stomach together so hard I would get headaches, tummy-aches and of course look ridiculous…

Also, I took the clothing that didn't fit and packed them away.
I didn't need that reminder every day.

Clothing is material (no pun intended), your health is much more important.
To give myself the breathing room to focus on my health and recovery.
It helped to buy myself a few beautiful pieces that made me feel great and made me smile.

I TOLD PEOPLE

Telling my husband was probably the easiest because he was my best friend and he witnessed the volcano erupt.
It was everyone else I found almost impossible.

I was paralysed with fear thinking about anyone I knew finding out that I had any issue with eating.
I mean, it wasn't half obvious. The constant fluctuation with my weight was probably a dead give-away… but I still found it embarrassing to have to tell anyone I didn't know how to eat!

I started a blog to help me get all my thoughts and learnings down, but I kept this a secret from everyone. Unless someone, somehow, stumbled across it online, my secret was safe.

When I stopped eating certain ingredients, some of my closest friends questioned me, I found it hard to not explain everything to them, but I also didn't know how to tell them.
It wasn't until about six months later, I told them.
Their reaction was fine. I didn't feel embarrassed or scared.
I had a massive hankering to help others, and I knew that eventually, I had to fight my fears and be open about everything.
There was no way I could keep it a secret and create a community where I helped others.

Somewhere along the way, I found my *'brave'* and invited my other friends and acquaintances to be part of the online community I had created where I was sharing my story.
That too didn't end up being as scary as I thought. Bit by bit, my *'scared'* was dissipating.

After a few months I also shared my story with other family members and as of today, the only person I haven't shared with is my stepdaughter.
I have held back from sharing anything with her because I haven't felt right sharing my issues as she is a growing young adult and has her own growing pains to deal with. Maybe this is the wrong approach, but I have been trying to protect her and give her less to worry about. I am sure at some stage I will share with her too as we are

very close. :)

The thought of telling people felt so shameful and embarrassing, but after ripping off the band-aid you realise nobody cares that much. Everyone has their own problems to deal with, and your story only gains a microsecond of airtime in their mind.

I wanted the world to see me as my authentic self, warts and all. I have nothing to hide and if I was to help others, I would have to be true to myself and the world.

MY LIFE LESSONS from ALL THE THINGS I DID RIGHT:

- I googled 'how to eat like a normal person'.
Google stuff. One thing leads to another. There is so much out there that could help you
- I read loads of books.
In the last two years I have read books such as The Year of Yes, Radical Self-Acceptance, The Power of Habit, Get your Sh*t Together, The 5 Second Rule, Thrive, Mindful Living, Intuitive Eating, Start with Why, Primal Blueprint, Grain Brain, Seven Habits of Highly Effective People, The Life-Changing Magic of Tidying up, Health at Every size, Embody, Food Junkies, The Life-Changing Magic of Not Giving a Fu*k, 21 Day Conscious Cleanse, Rising Strong and Why Diets Make Us Fat… amongst others.
Do you see how the books are not all about food and dieting? These books slowly came about as I uncovered different parts I needed to work on…
In your journey, you shouldn't just read the books I have

read, but instead, figure out where you want to start and your own learning journey will unfold.

• I found a page called 'The Moderation Movement'. These ladies speak all about self-love, they challenge everything you ever learned about health and are very in line with the Intuitive Eating & Health at Every Size approaches. This really made me never want to diet again.

• I went to a Naturopath.

I don't think I really needed this, but at the time I thought it was. Point being, follow what you feel you need to do. Going to the naturopath assisted me in uncovering that I needed to see a psychologist. Everything is part of the journey. Follow your gut.

• I went to a psychologist.

I did loads of research and found someone who specialised in my issues. She was a massive part of my recovery.

I even took my husband with me a few times. I wanted him to be part of the journey with me so he could understand my issue. I think it helped us as a couple too. Strike that. It helped us crap loads!

• I sat with my thoughts.

It is fine to go to a psychologist, but if you don't do some of your own questioning and self-exploration then you may not get where you need to be as quickly. I would literally sit in a room and ponder the situation and how I could fix it.

• I wrote stuff down.

I wrote heaps down. I challenged my thoughts, wrote more things down, brainstormed ideas regarding how I could 'heal' myself. I did not want to give up.

• Affirmations – I was kind to myself.

I read them, wrote them, coloured them in. I did
whatever it took.
I said nice, positive things to myself often.
- I practiced mindful, intuitive eating.
I ate slowly and concentrated on what I was eating.
Rather than eating as I was working or watching TV. I
concentrated on the experience of eating to ensure I
always felt good doing it.
- I fell and got back up again. Sometimes I didn't get up
    immediately. But I got up.
- I didn't want a life of eating disorders to be *my story*.
Even if I kept it to myself. I knew that was who I was. I
didn't want to look at myself that way anymore.
- I learned to take a compliment. Even if I didn't like it.

I have never given up on my dream to be the best
version of myself.
Not binging has been a by-product of getting my ducks
in a row and wanting it badly enough.
But first, I had to be OK with not being able to turn it off
like a tap. It took work. Once I realised this was the way
it had to be, I was OK with the journey.

Slow and steady has won the race.

Chapter 9 – Happily Ever After

We are all individuals.
I am guessing that if you have gotten this far, you may like what you have read? You may even want to make some changes in your own life.

One thing I have learned is that we are all individuals. I tried so many things on my journey, things I read in blogs or books, or courses.
What I have ended up with is my hybrid approach to health and happiness.

There was no program I could follow, no set way of recovery that works for everyone.

What worked for me, may not work for you. You may resonate with different practitioners.
You may think some of the stuff I did was airy-fairy.
I may think some of the stuff you do is airy-fairy.
It doesn't matter. As long as you choose things that resonate with you and make you feel like you are on the right track then it is right.

Following another person's version of a good life routine was never going to work for me. I needed to become my own life coach and design a life I loved.

If I didn't feel proud based on my values and ideas of what was right, I am wasn't living the life of my dreams...

YOU ARE THE MOST IMPORTANT PRACTITIONER OF YOUR RECOVERY

A session with a professional last an hour.
If my recovery didn't become my full-time focus, then one hour a fortnight would not help me much.

There were several times I went into a session only to come out thinking 'I don't feel any different or better'.

That's because one hour to explore your entire life sometimes isn't enough.

Often, I would have an epiphany or do extra journaling, exploring an issue we had discussed in session in my own time.
It was related to the session I had just had, but I had to put in the work myself to have the breakthroughs.

Much like going to a personal trainer.
Sure, it would be beneficial for you to have a one-hour session fortnightly with a personal trainer, but if you worked on your fitness a few times a week in your own time as well, you would reach your fitness goals faster with more consistency and depth.

Chapter 10 – Epilogue

IT'S NEVER OVER, BUT IT'S SO MUCH BETTER THAN YOU COULD EVER IMAGINE

A life of diets does not just go away.
I know that I must always be aware of when I am not in
self-care mode.
It happens, life happens, I will face challenging
moments in life that will send me to a place where self-
care may not be the priority.

My job will be to recognize these moments and do all I
can to restore my balance.

I am no longer naive to the fact that I have let dieting
rule my life and it will always be there (in the back seat)
to a certain extent.
But as each day goes by, I think about dieting less and
less. I rarely look at my body in disgust… except for
when I had a cold this week and got a fright when I
looked in the mirror! I looked like death warmed up.

My reflection is just my reflection. It isn't ugly. It just
is. And sometimes it is a good reflection, but when I
pass by a shop front and catch a glimpse I don't want to
crawl up in a corner and hide.

A few times I have had a realisation and thought 'Wow',
I am not doing *that* behaviour anymore, and I have not
done *that* for a long time, but truthfully, a small part of it
will probably always be there.
Even if it is just a subtle reminder.

It's nowhere near as bad as the feeling of having it
control my life like before.

And it's easy to deal with now I have the tools.

Knowing *it* is there, is different to *it* having full control over my life, like before.

Will Smith is not about to wipe my memory like in the movie 'Men in Black' and make me forget I was ever a dieter or hurt myself with food. And I don't want that.

I am stronger now.

AND FINALLY, TIME TO CELEBRATE!

For anyone on this journey, I must beg you, stress to you, pleeeead with you to celebrate your wins.

Celebrating wins is not like the wins you would celebrate when you were addicted to dieting.

I am pleased to say you need not wait to lose 5kg to treat yourself to that pedicure ever again!

I have celebrated when I have woken up in the morning realising that:

- My skin has looked amazing for the last month
- My clothes felt loose because I just knew how to eat on my own.
- I could do longer workouts
- I felt great for days on end
- I had confidence exuding from my body
- I had done things I would not normally do
- I realised I managed my eating in a healthy way
- I was doing activities I loved
- I was smiling during the day for no reason

The wins will look different to everyone, but a win is when you achieve the feeling you have been striving for. When you realise you are doing all that you love and managing life better than ever before, you have won.

Knowing I was not born this way, all-knowing and so wise for treating myself right is so much more rewarding.
I wasn't built this way. I made myself. I built this.
All by myself!

And you can too.